MED PG THRISSUR
AIIMS
Recall November 2017

Interactive post-publication support site for
MED PG THRISSUR AIIMS Recall November 2017
www.medpgthrissur.com

MED PG THRISSUR
AIIMS
Recall November 2017

Aswath Kumar MD FICOG
Professor
Department of Obstetrics and Gynecology
Jubilee Mission Medical College
Thrissur, Kerala, India

Bejohn Johnson Kunnath MS MCh (Ped Surg) Dip NB (Ped Surg)
Additional Professor
Department of Pediatric Surgery
Government Medical College
Thrissur, Kerala, India

Nidhish Chandra M MBBS
JIPMER 2017 Rank 1

Jereen M Peter MBBS
Junior Resident
Department of Radio-diagnosis
Amala Institute of Medical Sciences
Thrissur, Kerala, India

JAYPEE *The Health Sciences Publisher*
New Delhi | London | Panama

Jaypee Brothers Medical Publishers (P) Ltd

Headquarters

Jaypee Brothers Medical Publishers (P) Ltd
4838/24, Ansari Road, Daryaganj
New Delhi 110 002, India
Phone: +91-11-43574357
Fax: +91-11-43574314
Email: jaypee@jaypeebrothers.com

Overseas Offices

J.P. Medical Ltd
83 Victoria Street, London
SW1H 0HW (UK)
Phone: +44 20 3170 8910
Fax: +44 (0)20 3008 6180
Email: info@jpmedpub.com

Jaypee-Highlights Medical Publishers Inc
City of Knowledge, Bld. 235, 2nd Floor, Clayton
Panama City, Panama
Phone: +1 507-301-0496
Fax: +1 507-301-0499
Email: cservice@jphmedical.com

Jaypee Brothers Medical Publishers (P) Ltd
17/1-B Babar Road, Block-B, Shaymali
Mohammadpur, Dhaka-1207
Bangladesh
Mobile: +08801912003485
Email: jaypeedhaka@gmail.com

Jaypee Brothers Medical Publishers (P) Ltd
Bhotahity, Kathmandu
Nepal
Phone: +977-9741283608
Email: kathmandu@jaypeebrothers.com

Website: www.jaypeebrothers.com
Website: www.jaypeedigital.com

MED PG Thrissur AIIMS Recall November 2017

First Edition: **2018**

ISBN: 978-93-5270-359-3

Printed at: Samrat Offset Pvt. Ltd.

Preface

AIIMS Recall November 2017 is the fifth book of its kind from MED PG Thrissur. This book contains questions that are recalled by students.

Main features of this book are:

- Separate compilation of all images asked in AIIMS November 2017.
- Approximately 300 potential images and tables useful for last minute look.
- Exclusive chapter on Emergency Medicine.
- Topic-wise list of all questions asked in AIIMS November 2017.
- Tips to crack PG Entrance Examinations.

The notes which you have prepared for each subject should be the base for answering these questions. So, you should refer your notes for detailed explanation of questions. We have provided you with around 300 images, including tables that could be very useful for last minute revision. These images are also potential questions for upcoming NEET examinations as well. We have also included important points from each chapter which were not asked in AIIMS but can be asked for NEET.

The interactive section at *www.medpgthrissur.com* will address the queries from the readers. We would also encourage the readers to post their suggestions and opinions regarding the book.

Wishing all of you great successs in upcoming examinations.

Aswath Kumar
Bejohn Johnson Kunnath
Nidhish Chandra M
Jereen M Peter

Contents

Tips for Cracking PG Entrance Examinations

1. How to start preparation?

First thing in preparation is to know your examination. Knowing your examination includes:

A. Knowing how many questions, time, scheme of negative marking, how many questions to mark, how many questions to be correct, marks of previous year's topper, etc. If possible try to speak to one of your seniors who have cracked the examination and ask their opinion also. This gives you the right start for the race and avoid last minute doubts.

B. Another useful thing is to just go through at least three previous question papers before starting your preparation. There is no need to solve these in the beginning itself. This will help you concentrate more on the important topics and you will unknowingly be more attentive in class when your teacher go through these topics. It is just like having a route map before going to sea.

2. How many hours to study?

I think quality is more important than quantity. Make time tables for each subject and try to finish them in time. Sometimes, you may not be able to complete in time, but still move forward. Identify the best time, method and atmosphere to study during the initial phase itself so that during the last phase of preparation you can be so fast.

3. What should be the strategy for studying?

Making notes is the most important step in studying. After making notes, do tests regularly and identify the missing points and add them onto your notes. Tests also gives you an analysis of our performance, time management and what are your weak areas.

4. How to prepare for AIIMS?

For all examinations, whether it be institute or NEET PG, notes should be your strongest asset. So, finish notes first, then spend time on five previous papers and concentrate more on solution part as topic repeats are nowadays asked in AIIMS. (Sometimes, you may get direct question repeats also). Analyze the pattern of questions asked and anticipate questions. For example, last time they asked images of instruments used in orthopedics and ophthalmology, and this time they asked obstetrics and gynecology instruments, so we can anticipate more practical-based questions in the following papers also. The pattern of image-based questions are still continuing and emergency medicine has gained a great significance in the recent years and hopefully will continue.

5. How to prepare for JIPMER?

Again, notes are the first and most important tool. Unlike AIIMS, the number of images are very less. Doing about five previous papers is a must because direct question repeats are more for JIPMER. By doing this, we also get to know the favourite topics frequently asked (genetic mutations, newer monoclonal antibodies, anticancer drugs, drugs for irritable bowel syndrome, calculation-based questions in physiology, SPM). Always try to attempt more questions in JIPMER (close to 235), because as the number of seats are less, you need to have a very good rank to get the seat of your choice. Comparing to AIIMS, you can make more mistakes in JIPMER (try not to make, if possible). I had around 165 correct answers but had made around 85 wrong. So, I feel that it is not the number of wrong answers that matters, but the number of correct responses.

6. How to prepare for NEET PG?

Again notes are the key. Comparing to AIIMS and JIPMER, the questions will be almost basic concepts which would be there in your notes. So, it is always very important to expand your notes by adding your mistakes that you have committed in the tests. Number of images will be less compared to AIIMS, but there can be few.

7. What to study one month before the examination?

Never try to learn anything new during the last one month. Try to finish your notes at the earliest and concentrate on the examination you are more interested and be thorough with the questions and the topics asked in that examination. Always try to read the examiner's mind by anticipating the next year's questions.

8. What to do one week before the examination?

Try to revise your notes of all the 19 subjects during the last week (if not possible, at least the important topics) as this gives you a great deal of confidence during examination to attempt all subjects. Always focus on rectifying mistakes that you made during the examinations you wrote earlier. During the last week, also go through all the images you have seen before.

9. What to do one day before the examination?

Relax and focus on the most volatile areas in which you are not confident. Do not listen to anyone else. Just focus on your weak areas, not others weak area. Pray to God and talk to your parents and teachers, get their blessings and sleep well on the day before.

10. What to do at the time of examination?

Have a silent prayer before the examination and write the examination as if you should get the first rank. This makes sure that you do not take any question lightly and give your 100%. There may be some difficult questions in examinations, sometimes they may come in a row, so do not feel dejected. See the questions one by one, if you do not know the answer, just mark it for review. Do not keep the answers which you know to be marked at the end. If time is short, you may fail to save these.

Trust in God and keep moving, you will reach there.

ALL THE BEST!!!!

Nidhish Chandra M
(Rank 1, JIPMER November 2017 Session)

Topic-wise List of Questions Asked in AIIMS November 2017

Anatomy

1. Examples of joint type
2. Development of heart
3. Histology of cardiac muscle
4. Shape of trapezius
5. Muscles of mastication
6. Root value of reflexes
7. Identifying lateral semicircular canal
8. Brainstem section showing cranial nerves
9. Anatomy of PCL of knee
10. Structures passing through diaphragm
11. Development and growth of paranasal sinuses
12. Abducens nerve palsy
13. Holocrine glands histology
14. Gray and white rami communicans
15. Locations of dense irregular collagen
16. Anatomy of perineal body
17. Kiesselbach plexus
18. Ossification of carpal bones
19. Commissural fibers of white matter

Physiology

1. Basal electric rhythm
2. Cardiac reflexes
3. Stages of sleep
4. Diurnal variation of growth hormone secretion
5. Feed forward control system
6. Regulation of GFR
7. Hysteresis loop of inspiration and expiration
8. Refractory period
9. Resting membrane potential
10. Susceptibility of nerve fiber to LA

Pathology

1. Storage period of blood with various anticoagulants
2. Intrinsic and extrinsic pathway of coagulation

3. Vacutainers, color coding and anticoagulant used
4. HPE of schwannoma
5. Peripheral smear of thalassemia
6. Correct order of collecting blood from patient
7. Parameters altered in iron deficiency anemia
8. HER2/new and FISH
9. HPE of FB aspiration pneumonia
10. Cells of origin of leukemia
11. Chloroma
12. Approach to polycythemia
13. HPE of squamous cell carcinoma esophagus
14. Aschoff bodies
15. Fixatives used in pathology
16. Tumor markers in ovarian malignancies
17. Type of collagen seen in renal basement membrane

Biochemistry

1. Glycogen storage disorder
2. Post-translational modification
3. Glucosamine uses
4. Vitamins functioning as coenzymes
5. Biochemical test for ketone body, sugar and proteins
6. DNA repair and associated conditions
7. Proteins involved in iron metabolism
8. Dried blood drop test in an infant

Microbiology

1. Relapse and recrudescence in malaria
2. Dimorphic fungus
3. Diagnosis of neonatal CMV
4. Blood spill disinfection
5. 1,3 beta-D glucose assay
6. Lipoarabinomannan (LAM) assay
7. Diagnosis of *Cl. difficile* infection
8. Viral hemorrhagic fever in India
9. Types of flagella
10. Replication of hepatitis B
11. Fecal stain specimen
12. Image of *Aspergillus*
13. Hand–foot–mouth disease
14. Sclerotic bodies in chromoblastomycosis

Forensic Medicine and Toxicology

1. PM appearance in throttling
2. Declarations
3. Cocaine and LSD
4. Termination of pregnancy
5. Appearance of rigor mortis
6. Atropine as antidote
7. Specimen collecting in firearm injury
8. McNaughten's rule
9. As poisoning

Pharmacology

1. Mechanism of action of antibiotics
2. Antihypertensives and contraindications
3. MOA of steroid in a/c asthma
4. Agonist and antagonist of opioids
5. Induction of anesthesia
6. Receptors in sympathetic system
7. Calculation-based problem
8. Treatment of diarrhea
9. DOC for scrub typhus
10. Management of hyperkalemia
11. Response of epinephrine in septic shock
12. Specific side effects of OHA
13. Examples of placebo
14. Syndromic approach in STD
15. Uses of bromocriptine
16. Dose of epinephrine in anaphylactic shock
17. Treatment of motion sickness
18. Biofilm mechanism of resistance
19. Precautions for a lactating mother
20. Specific side effect of antitubercular drugs
21. MOA of antianginal
22. Newer hypolipidemic agents
23. Drugs for acute rejection after transplant
24. Newer drugs for breast cancer

Obstetrics and Gynecology

1. Clinical examination of a pregnant women
2. Instruments used in obstetrics and gynecology
3. Partogram

4. HPV vaccine
5. Calculation of EDD from LMP
6. Stages of labor
7. Treatment of endometrial hyperplasia
8. Emergency contraception
9. Hypogonadotropic hypogonadism
10. Turner's syndrome
11. Extracalorie requirement in pregnancy
12. Evaluation of postcoital bleeding

Surgery

1. Marker of fluid resuscitation in trauma
2. Modified shock index
3. Color coding of cannula
4. Primary and secondary survey in trauma
5. Foley's catheter
6. Preoperative surgical check list
7. Balanced resuscitation
8. Gallbladder pathology
9. Desmoid tumor
10. Pain at lumbar region
11. ICD tube functioning
12. Follow up of renal laceration and urinoma
13. Management of renal calculus
14. Tumor lysis syndrome
15. Length of NG tube insertion
16. Blister formation in burns
17. Glasgow coma scale

Orthopedics

1. Proximal humerus fracture
2. Sprengel's deformity and Klippel-Feil syndrome
3. GA classification of open fracture
4. Hoover's test
5. Fracture scaphoid

Social and Preventive Medicine

1. Ordinal scale of measurement
2. Unvaccinated child
3. Crude birth rate and number of ANC units
4. Mid-day meal

5. Alpha error
6. Triage in trauma
7. Vaccine vial monitoring
8. Sensitivity and specificity
9. Absolute and relative risk calculation

Ophthalmology

1. Refractory errors
2. Pterygium
3. Management of endophthalmitis
4. Nonproliferative diabetic retinopathy
5. Staphyloma
6. Lacrimal gland tumor

Skin

1. Hutchinson's triad
2. Blister in burns
3. Fixed-drug eruption
4. Desmosomes—location in histology slide

Radiology

1. DSA image of internal carotid artery
2. Investigation of choice in SAH
3. Management of large cerebral infarct with midline shift
4. Carcinoids
5. Spontaneous pneumothorax—chest X-ray

Medicine

1. Steps of basic life support
2. ECG interpretation
3. Blood transfusion complication
4. Menke's disease
5. Necrobiosis diabeticorum
6. Dulling of first heart sound in mitral stenosis
7. Serum ascites albumin gradient
8. High anion gap and normal anion gap metabolic acidosis
9. Evaluation of SVC syndrome
10. Murmurs
11. Management of SVT
12. CSF analysis

13. Hepatitis B and progression of cancer
14. Ice pack test in myasthenia gravis

Ear, nose and throat

1. Semicircular canal
2. CSF rhinorrhea
3. Growth of sinuses
4. Noise-induced hearing loss
5. Recurrent laryngeal nerve palsy

Anesthesia

1. Management of intubated patient
2. Preanesthetic medications
3. Preoxygenation in GA

Pediatrics

1. Management of neonatal jaundice
2. Apgar source (asked twice)
3. Developmental delay

Psychiatry

1. Acute side effects of antipsychotics
2. Delusion
3. Dysthymia
4. Collecting history of a psychiatric patient from an informant
5. Capgras syndrome
6. Immediate memory test

Images Asked in AIIMS November 2017

Anatomy

Q. 1

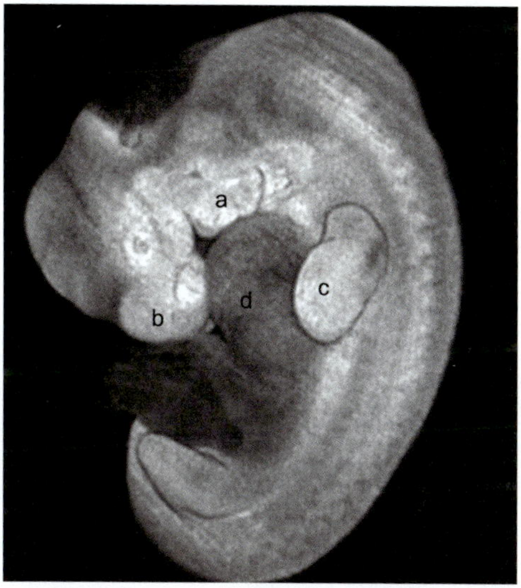

Q. 2

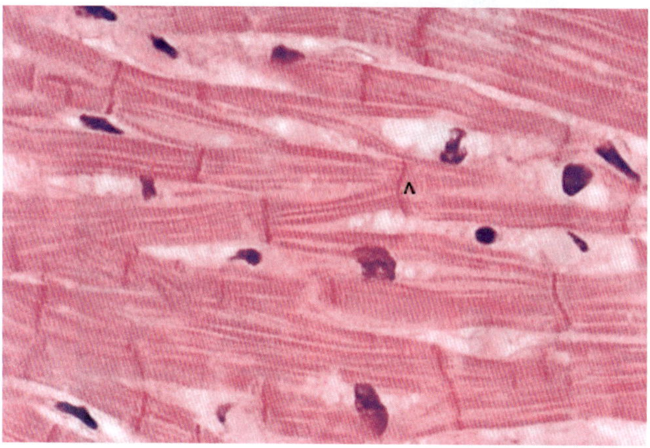

Q. 4

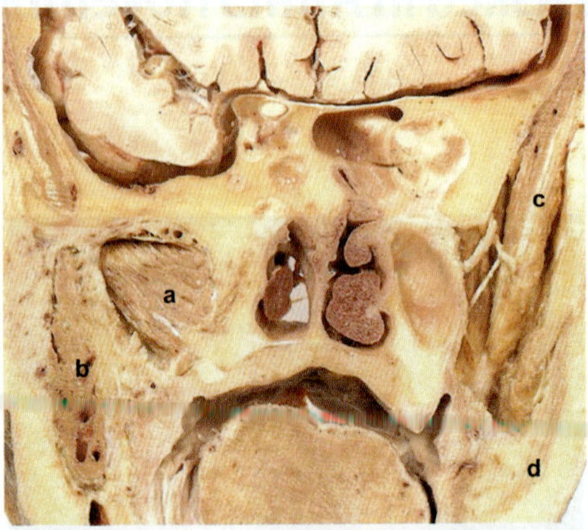

Q. 6

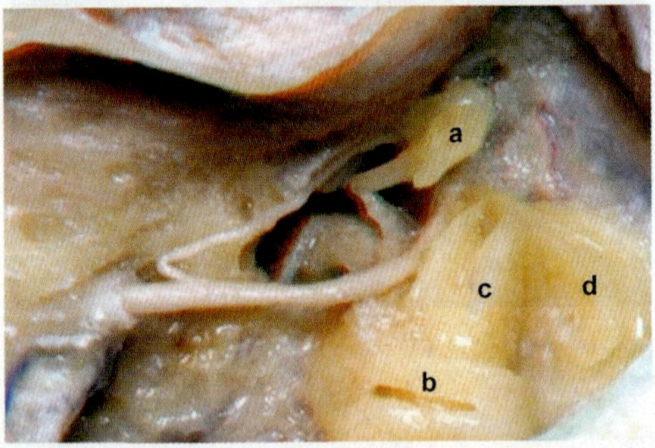

Q. 7

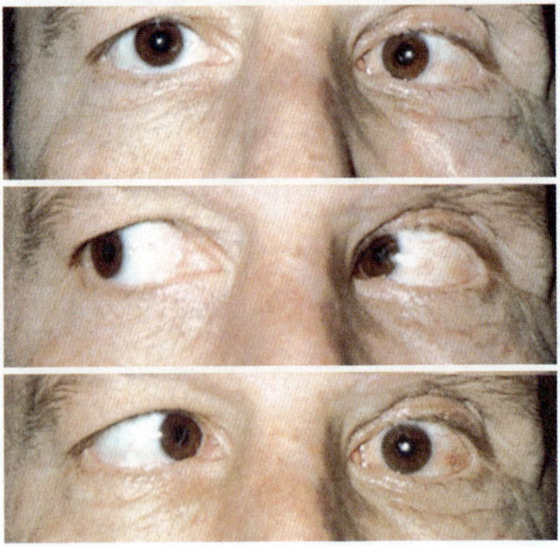

Q. 11

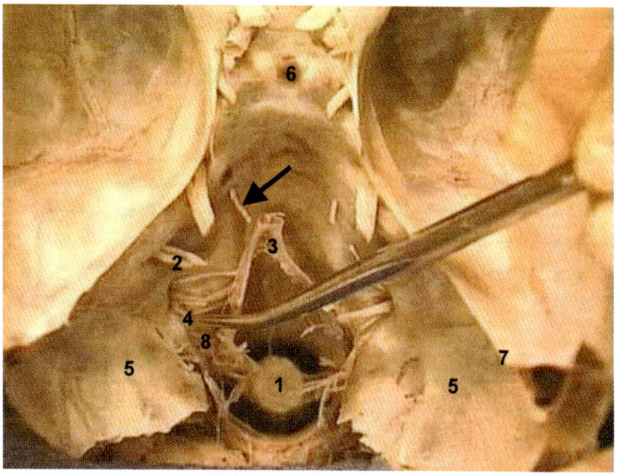

Q. 12

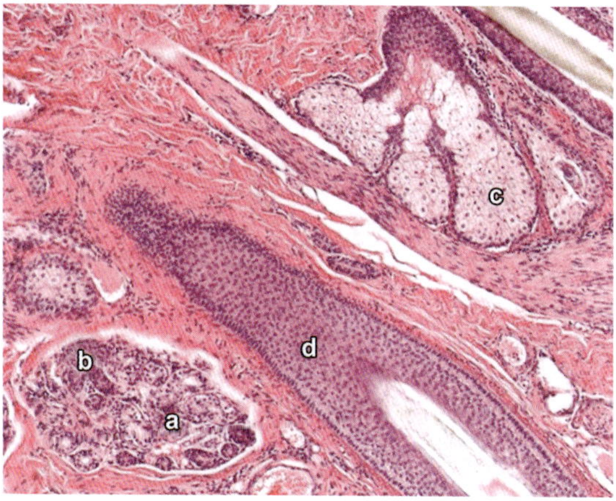

Q. 18

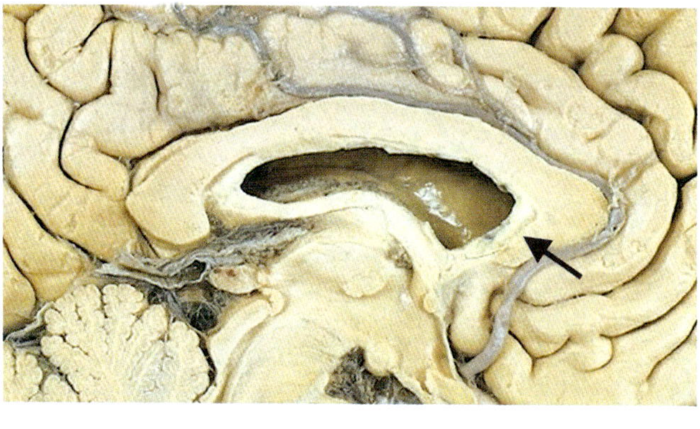

Physiology

Q. 3

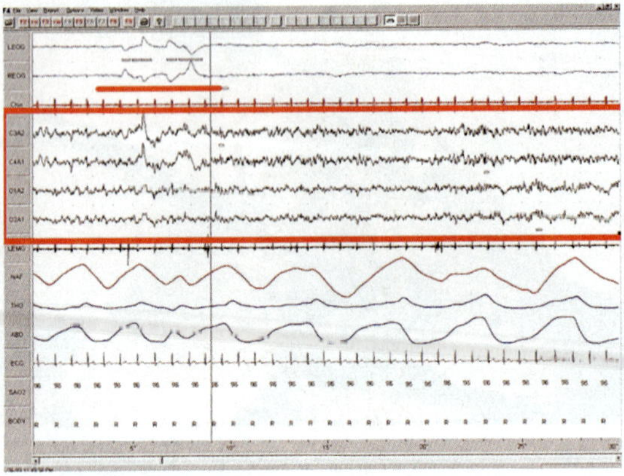

Q. 4

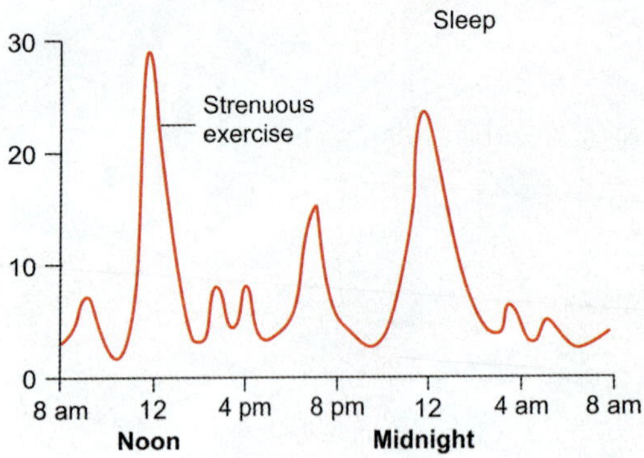

Q. 6

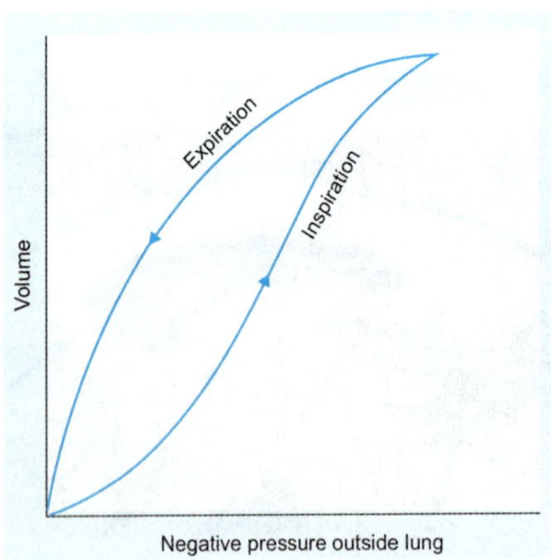

Biochemistry

Q. 5

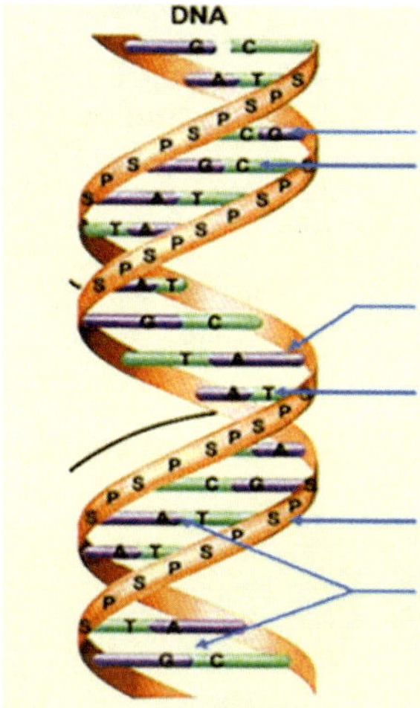

Q. 6

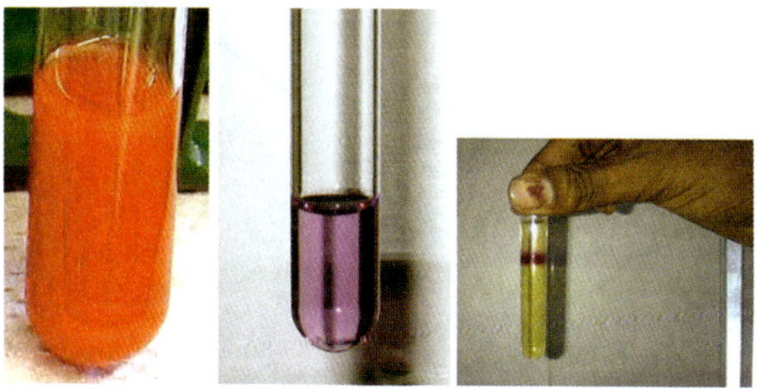

Pathology

Q. 4

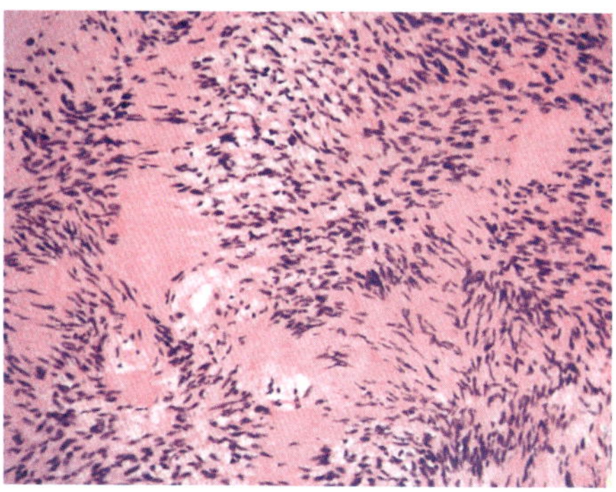

Q. 5

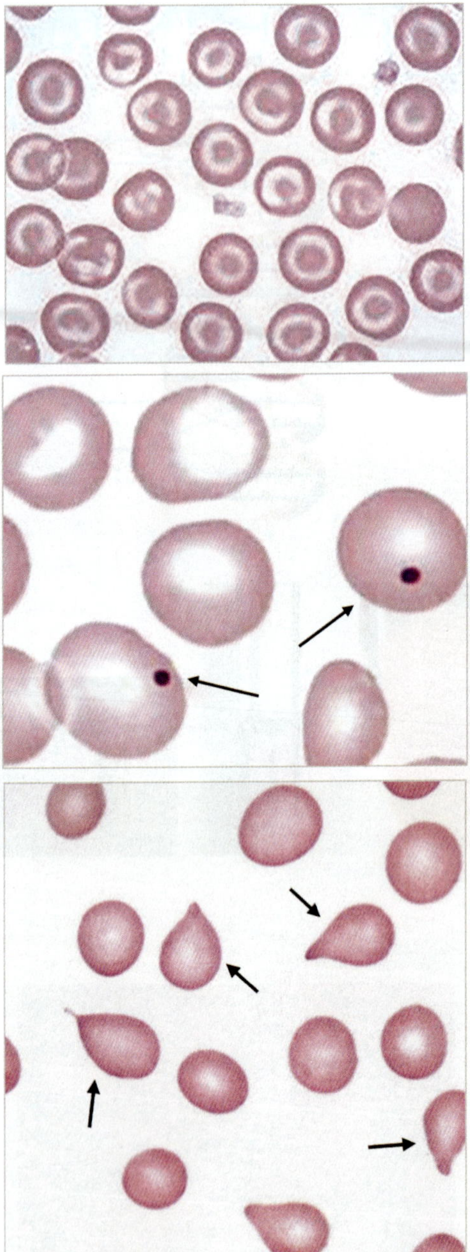

Q. 9

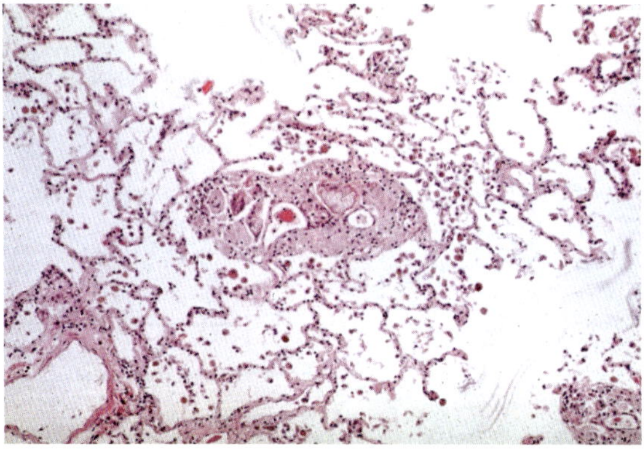

Q. 13

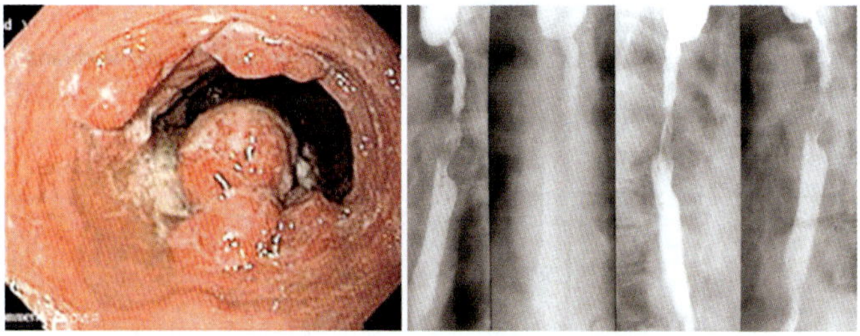

Q. 14

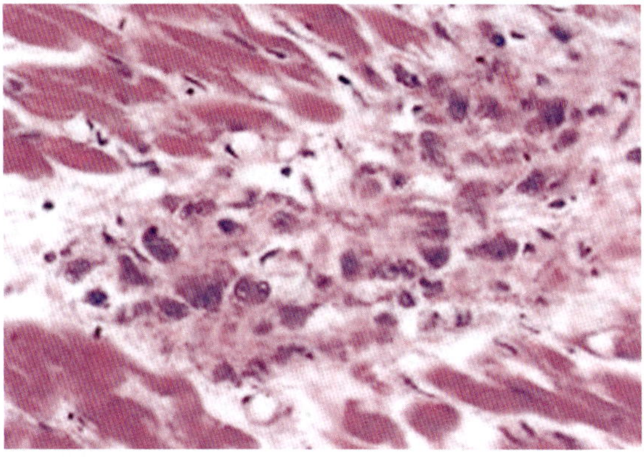

Microbiology

Q. 9

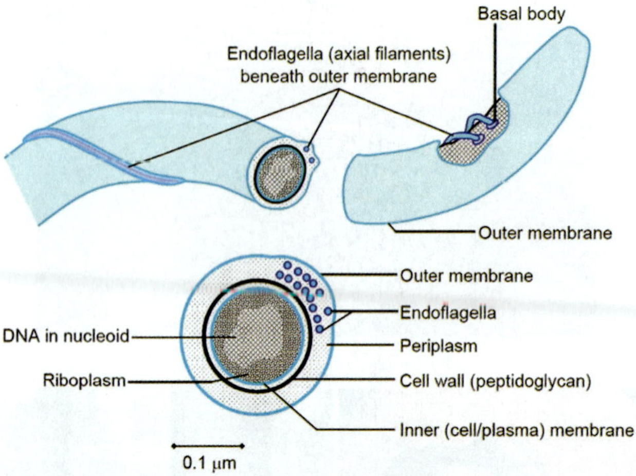

Q. 10

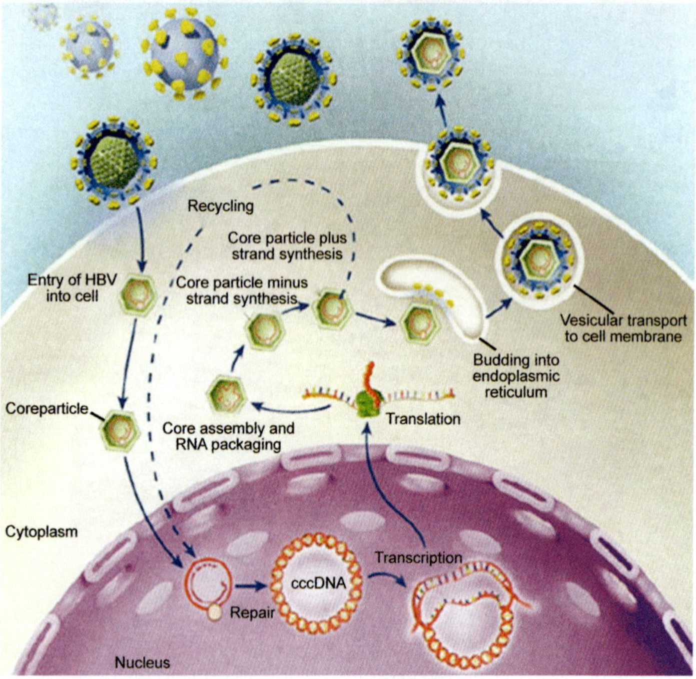

Q.11

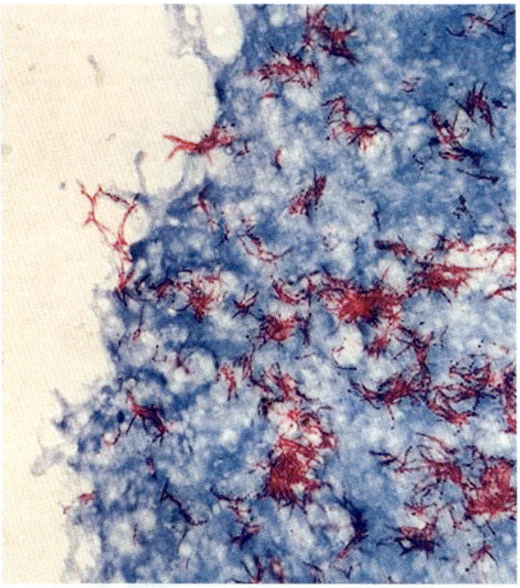

Q. 12

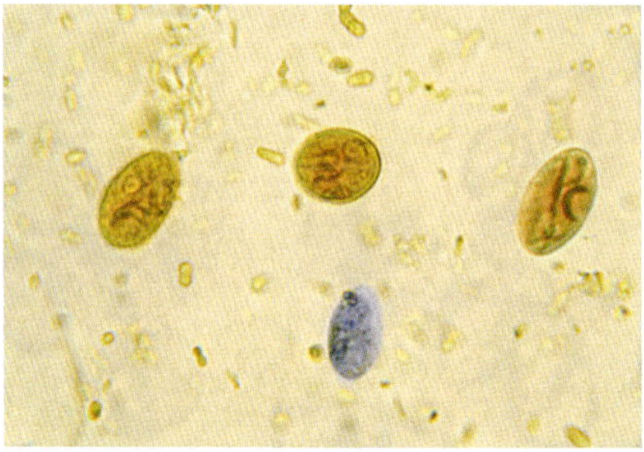

Q. 13

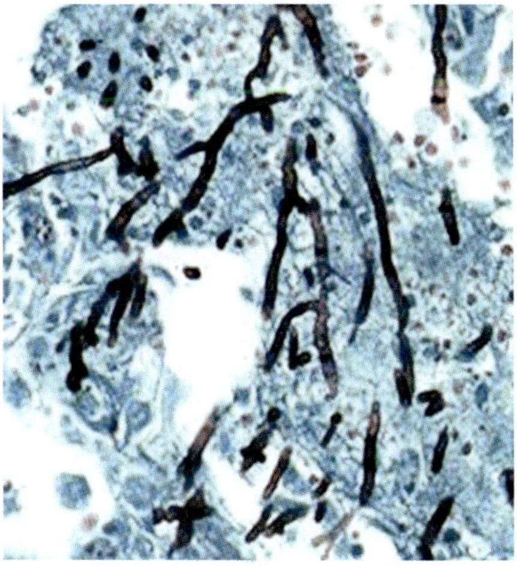

Q. 14

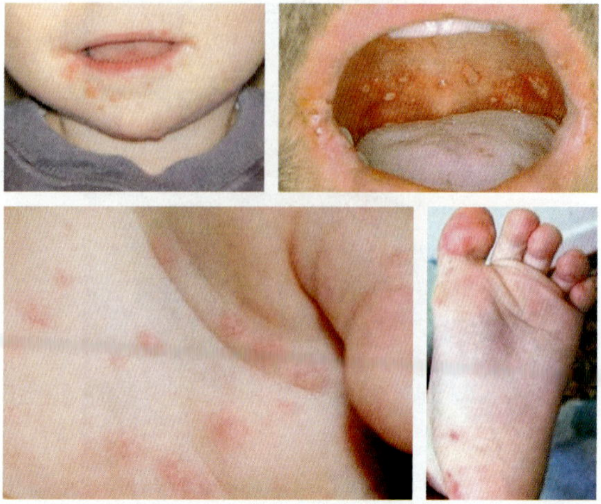

Q. 15

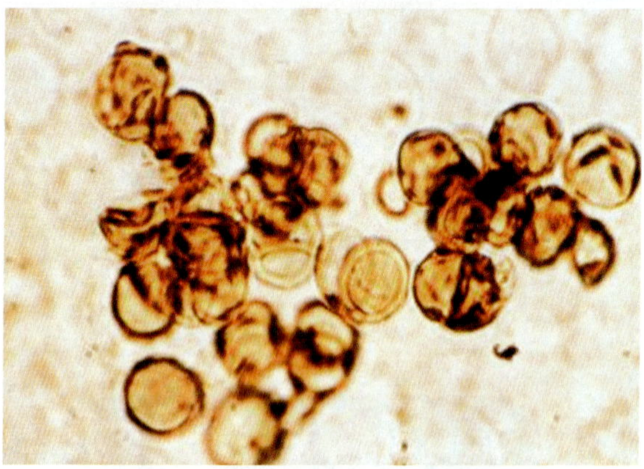

Forensic Medicine and Toxicology

Q. 1

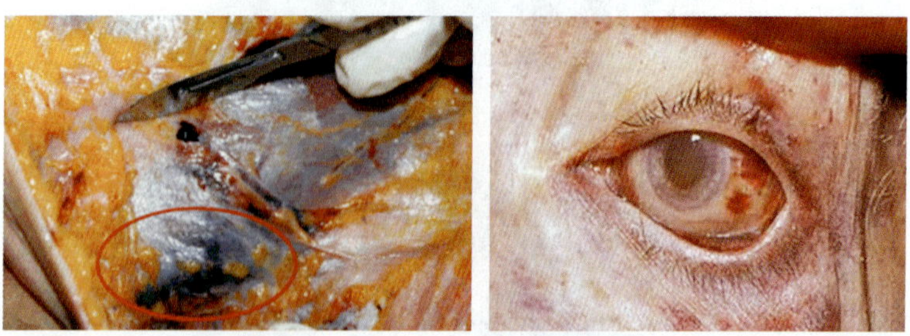

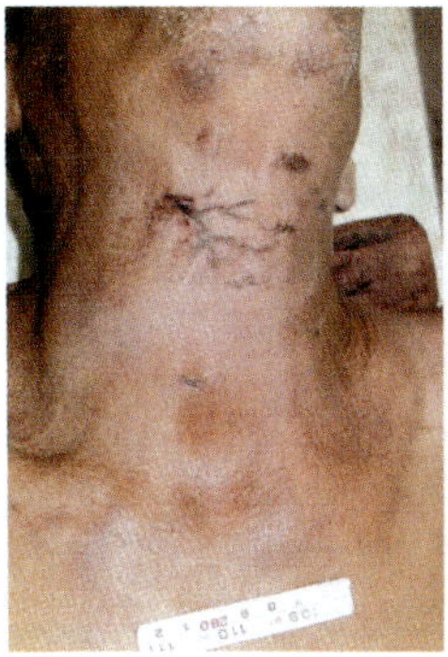

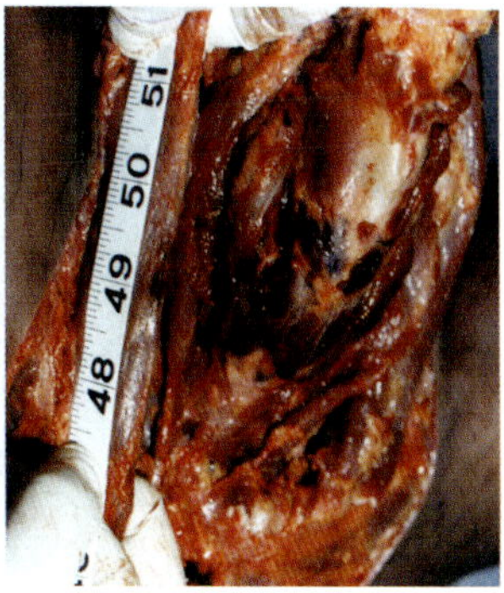

Obstetrics and Gynecology

Q. 1

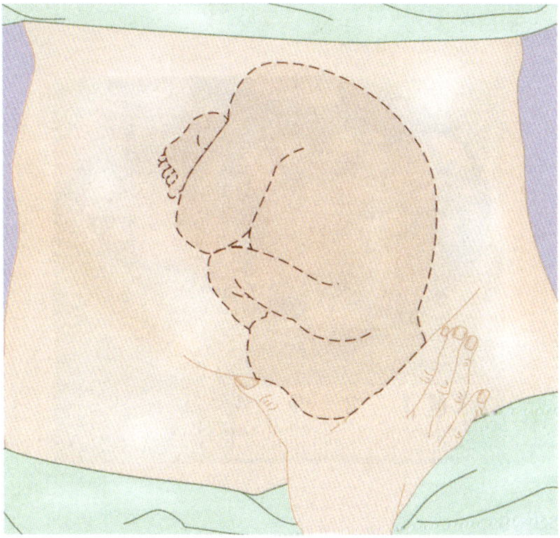

Q. 2

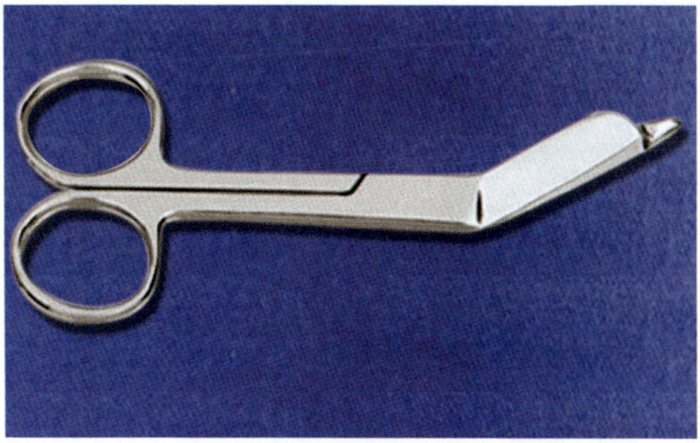

Q. 3

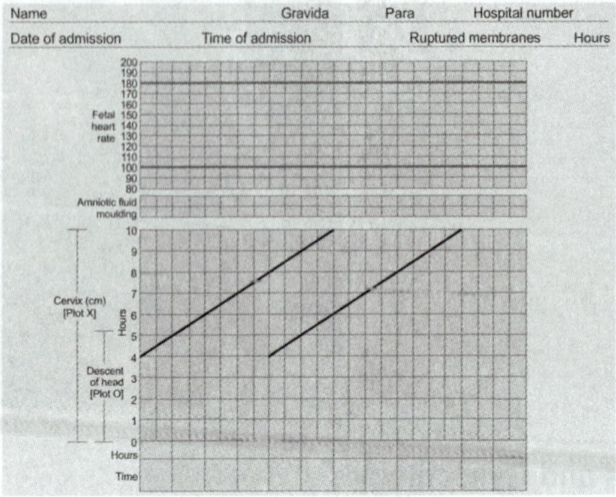

Surgery

Q. 7

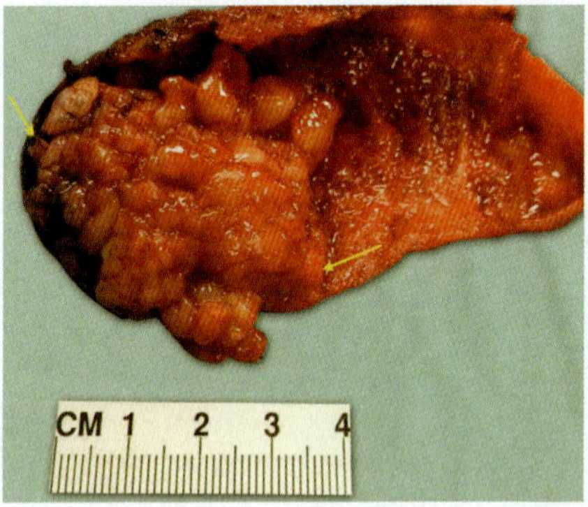

Orthopedics

Q. 2

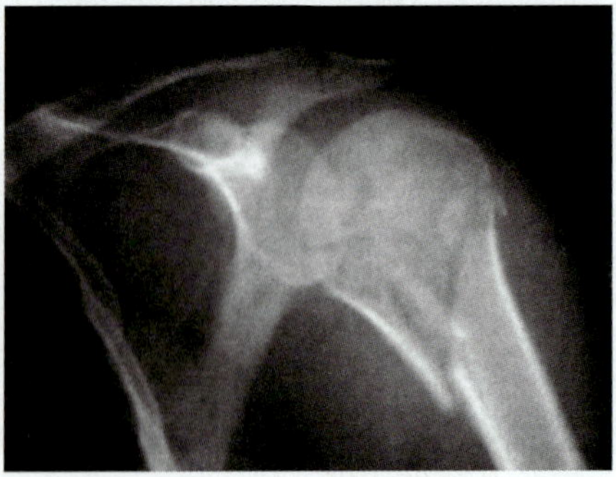

Q. 6

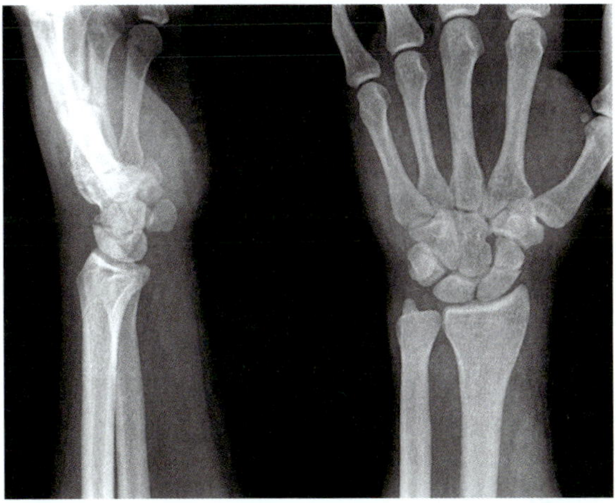

Ophthalmology

Q. 1

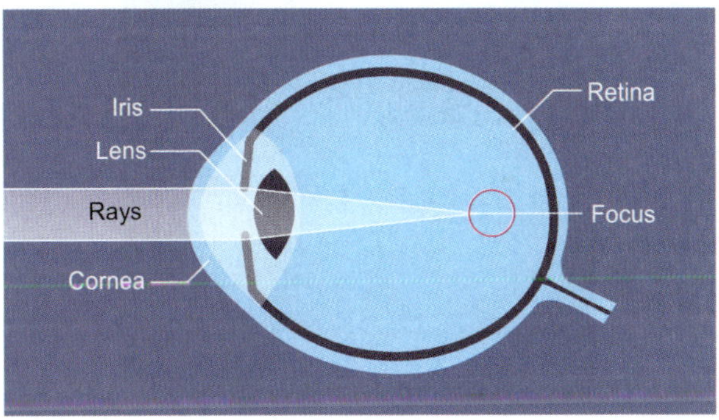

Q. 2

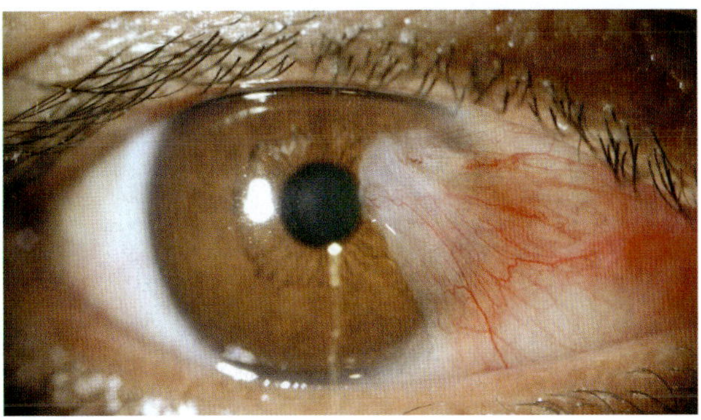

Q. 4

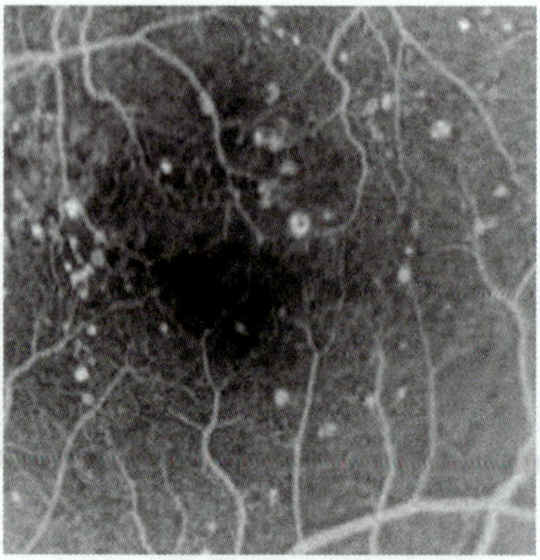

Dermatology

Q. 2

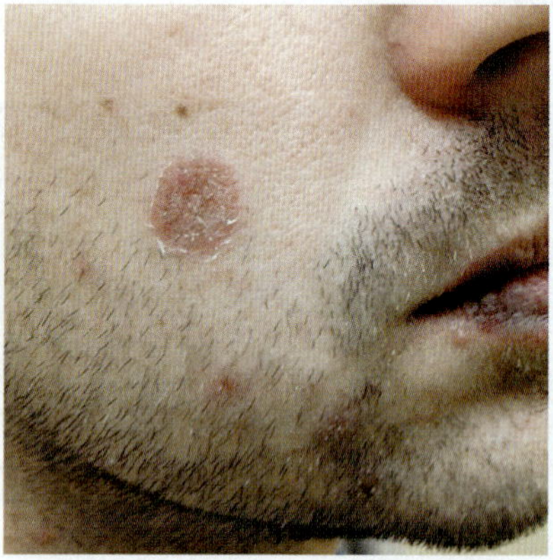

Q. 3

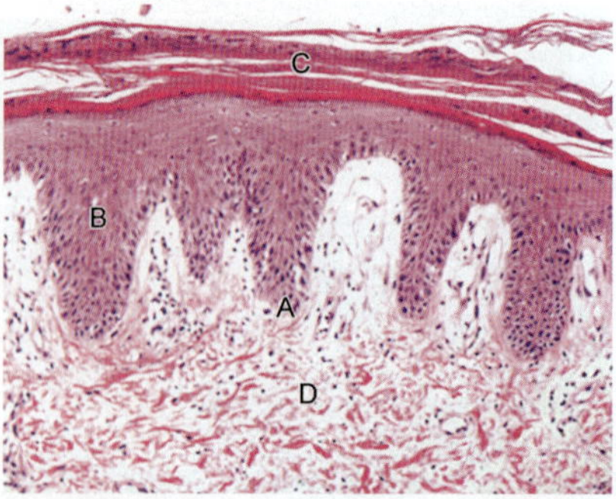

Radiology

Q. 1

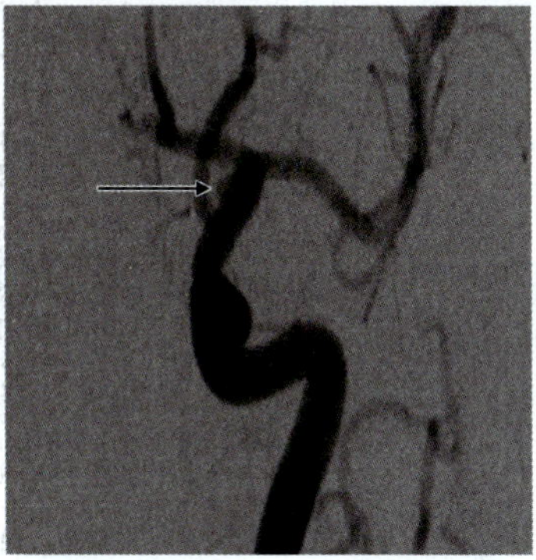

Medicine

Q. 1

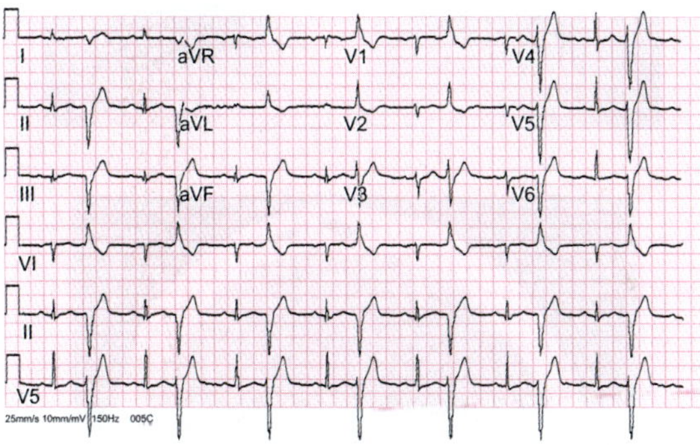

Q. 5

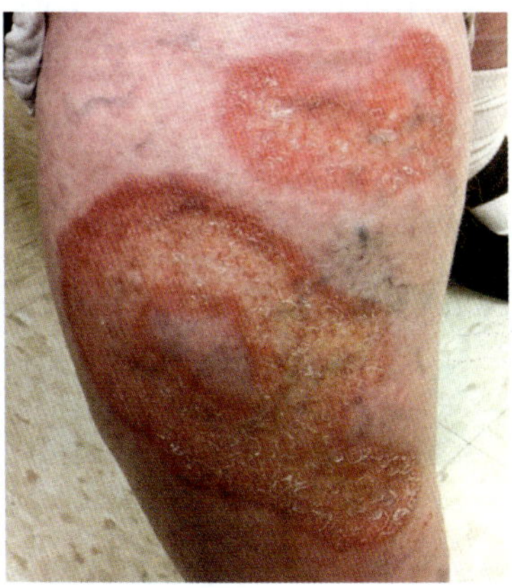

Q. 12

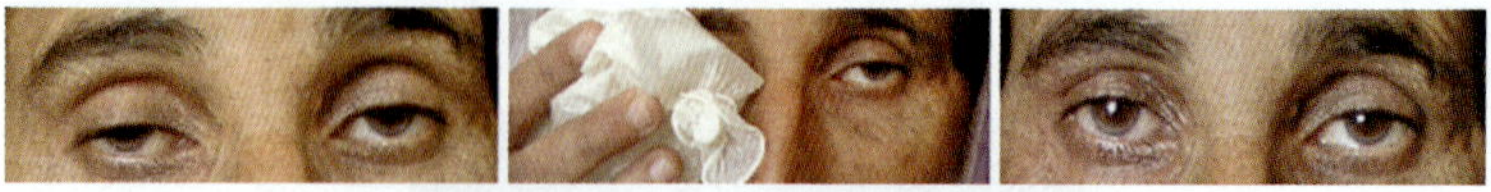

Emergency Medicine

Q. 3

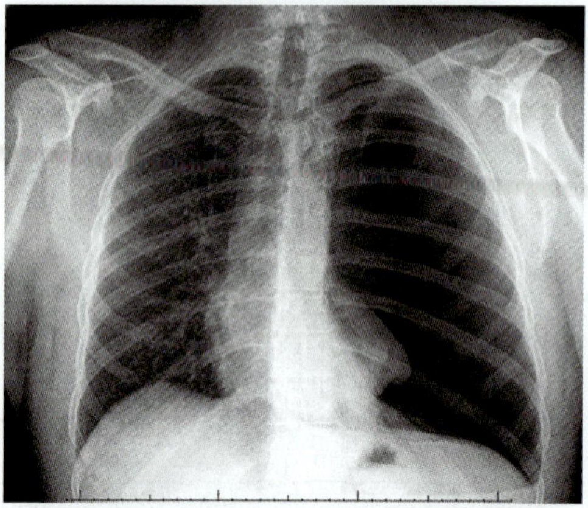

Q. 5

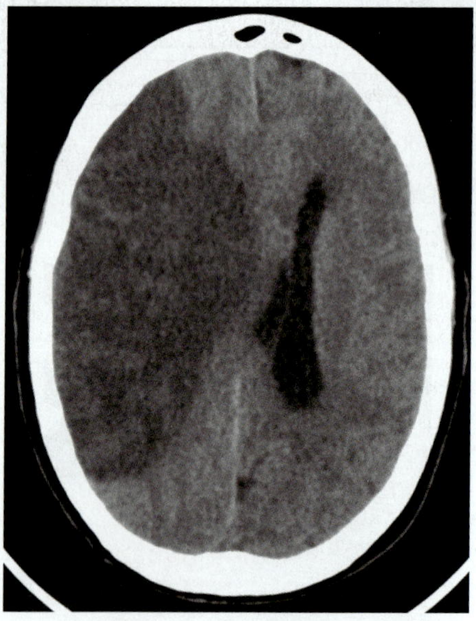

1

CHAPTER

Anatomy

1. Development of heart is from which of the following:

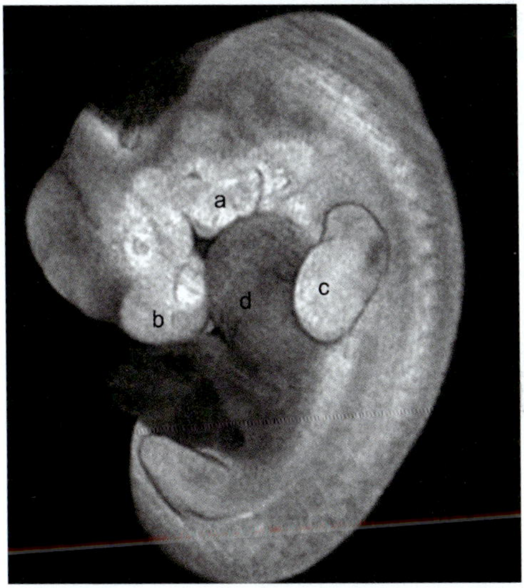

A. Pharyngeal arches B. Forebrain
C. Upper limb D. Heart

ANS. **D**

There has been a rising trend of asking embryology images in AIIMS. May session had asked the development of nucleus pulposus (Answer was notochord).

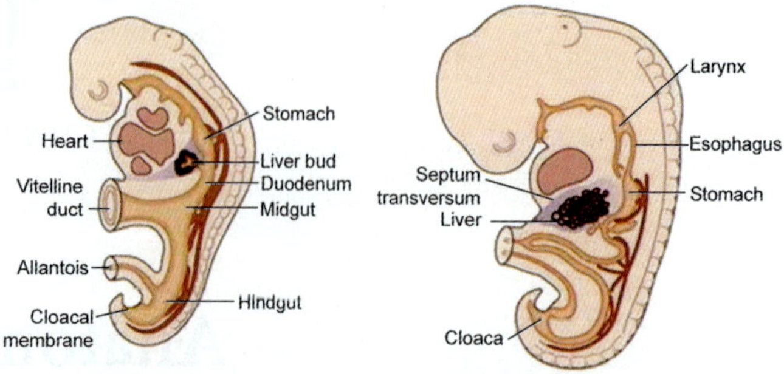

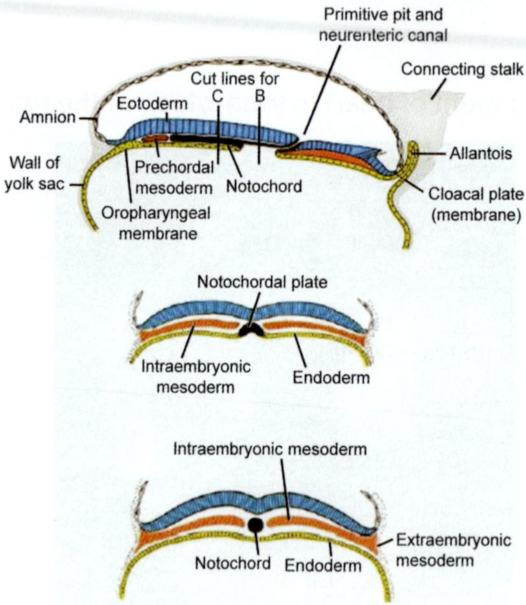

Development of cerebral cortex

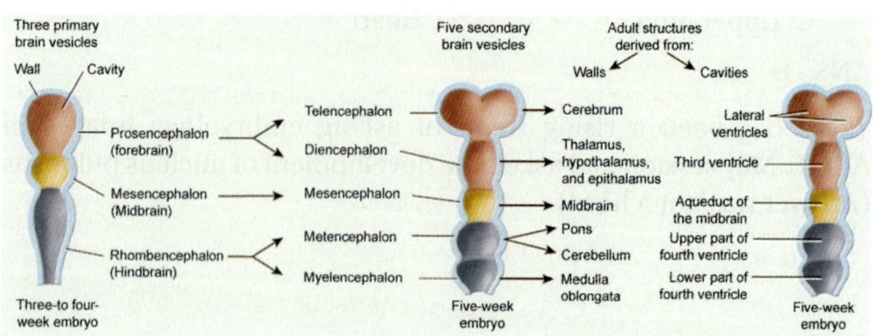

Development of palate and anomalies of it

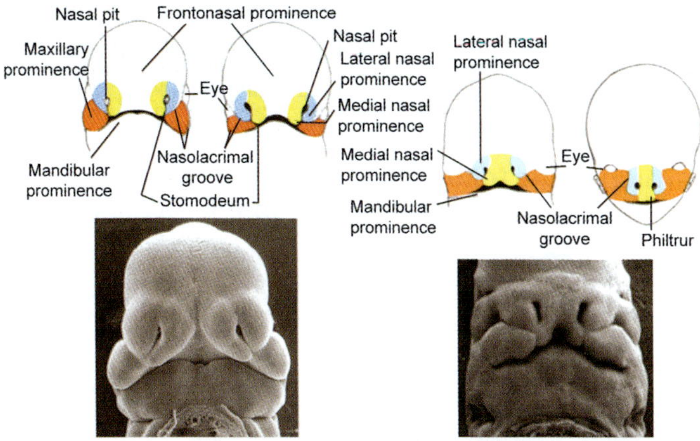

- Midline cleft lip: Due to non-fusion of 2 median nasal process
- Harelip (not midline): Due to non-fusion of medial nasal process and maxillary process
- Oblique facial cleft: Non-fusion of maxillary and lateral nasal process

Pharyngeal pouch and cleft

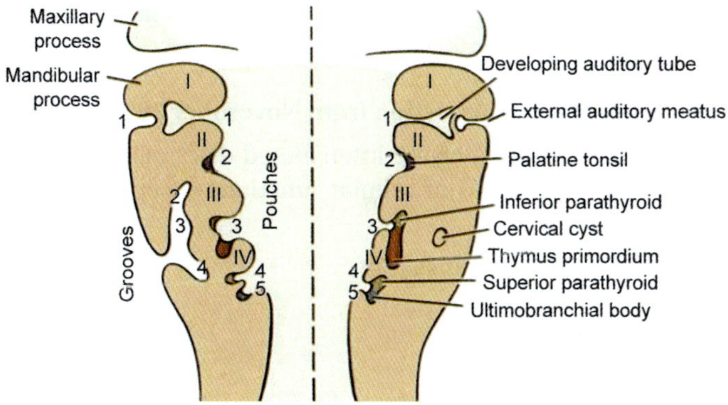

Another important area is remnants of various structures

Right umbilical vein	Disappears
Left umbilical vein	Ligamentum teres
Proximal part of umbilical artery	Superior vesical artery
Distal part of umbilical artery	Lateral umbilical ligament

Ductus arteriosus	Ligamentum arteriosum
Ductus venosus	Ligamentum venosum
Urachus	Median umbilical ligament
Obliterated umbilical artery	Medial umbilical fold
Inferior epigastric artery	Lateral umbilical fold

2. Which of the following junctional complexes are not seen in the area marked as A in the given slide?

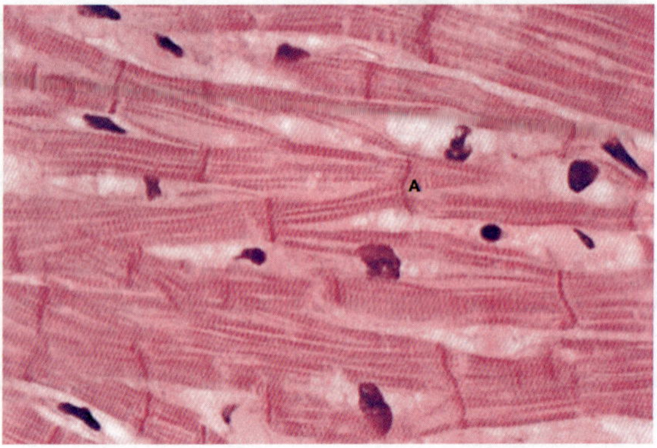

A. Gap junction
B. Zona occludens
C. Fascia adherens
D. Macula adherens

ANS. **B**

This is a direct repeat question from November 2016.

The given diagram is showing intercalated discs of cardiac muscle, which contains all types of cellular junctions except tight junction (zona occludens).

So, the cardiac muscle consists of:

1. Gap junctions
2. Fascia adherens
3. Macula adherens

Intercalated disc is a junctional complex between neighboring cells in the cardiac muscle cells. The interdigitating transverse parts of the intercalated disc form a fascia adherens, with numerous desmosomes.

Gap junctions are found in the longitudinal parts of the disc.

Another important point in this regard is the various types of adhesive contacts:

1. Zona adherens: These are continuous zones of adhesion present parallel and just basal to tight junction in epithelia. This area has high concentration of cadherins.

(Remember, cadherin is responsible for metastasis of tumor cells and E-cadherin mutation is seen in lobular carcinoma breast and diffuse gastric carcinoma)

2. Desmosomes: These are strongly seen in areas of intercellular contact. Desmosomes form strong anchorage points between cells subject to mechanical stress.

(This time they had given a histology of skin and asked to mark the area with highest concentration of desmosomes. So this area of cellular adhesions are very important).

3. Hemidesmosome: These are anchoring junctions between bases of epithelial cells and basal lamina.

Hemidesmosomes use integrin as adhesion molecules whereas desmosomes use cadherins.

3. What is the shape of trapezius muscle?

A. Quadrangular C. Strap
B. Triangular D. Fusiform

ANS. **B**

The **trapezius** is a flat. **Triangular muscle**, covering the upper and back part of the neck and shoulders (Grays anatomy).

Origin: Spinous process of C7, external occipital protuberance, medial third of superior nuchal line and ligamentum nuchae.

Insertion: Posterior border of lateral third of clavicle.

Nerve supply: Spinal accessory nerve.

Actions: Rotation, retraction, elevation and depression of scapula.

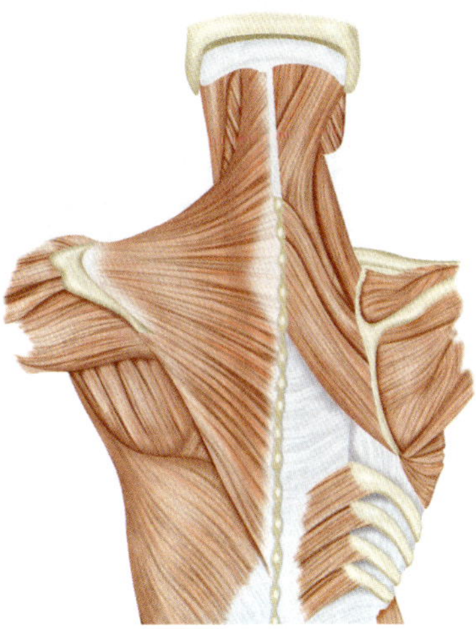

4. Which of the following muscle helps in opening of jaw?

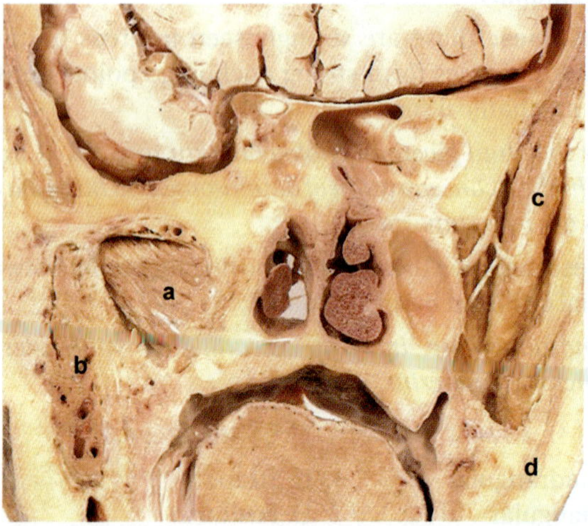

A. a C. c
B. b D. d

ANS. **A**

a: Lateral pterygoid (opening and protraction)
b: Masseter (closing)
c: Temporalis (closing and retraction)
d: Buccinator (cheek inflation)

This is a topic repeat from AIIMS November 2015. The question asked was to mark lateral pterygoid.

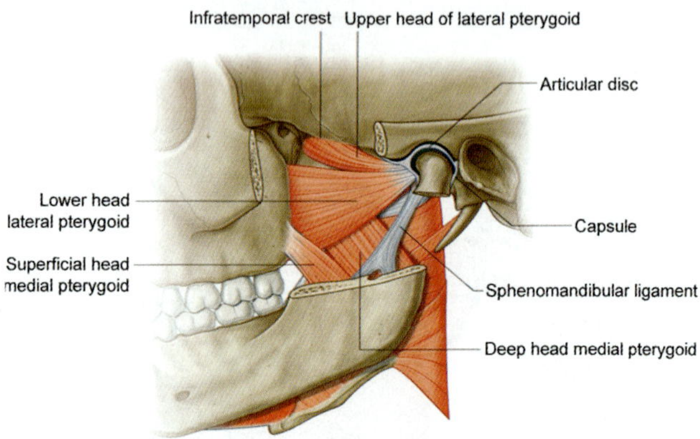

Movements of mandible				
Protraction	*Retraction*	*Depression*	*Elevation*	*Side to side*
• Lateral pterygoid • Medial pterygoid	Posterior fibers of temporalis	• Lateral pterygoid • Digastric • Geniohyoid • Myelohyoid	• Masseter • Medial pterygoid • Temporalis	• Lateral pterygoid • Medial pterygoid

5. Root value of cremastric reflex?

A. L1-L2 B. L2-L3 C. S1-S2 D. L4-L5

ANS. **A**

Important dermatomes

C1-No sensory supply
C2-Occiput
C5-Shoulder region (deltoid)
C7-Middle finger area
T2/T3-Axilla
T7-Epigastrium
T10-Umblicus
T12-Pubic symphysis
L3-Knee
L5-Outer aspect of leg
S1-Lateral aspect of sole (walking on S1)
S3, S4, S5-Around the anus (sitting on S3,4,5)

Important spinal segments to remember

C5-Abduction of shoulder
C6-Flexion of elbow
C7-Extension of elbow
C8-Wrist flexion and extension
T1-Small muscles of hand
L1-Flexion of hip
L2-Adduction of hip
L3-Extension of knee
L4-Dorsiflexion of ankle and inversion of foot
L5-Eversion of foot
S1-Plantar flexion of ankle

S2, 3-Small muscles of foot
L4, L5-Abduction of hip
L5, S1-Extension of hip and flexion of knee
L5-Extensor digitorum hallucis
S1-Flexor digitorum hallucis

Root value of reflexes

Superficial reflexes

Conjunctival and corneal reflex: Trigeminal (ophthalmic division)
Superficial abdominal reflex: T7-T12 spinal segments
Anal reflex: S2, 3, 4
Bulbocavernous reflex: S3, 4 (pudendal nerve)
Plantar reflex: L5, S1
Cremastric reflex: L1, L2 (ilioinguinal nerve—afferent and genitofemoral nerve—efferent).

Deep reflexes

Biceps reflex: C5, 6 (musculocutaneous nerve)
Supinator reflex: C5, 6 (radial nerve)
Triceps reflex: C6, 7 (radial nerve)
Knee jerk: L2 ,3, 4 (femoral nerve)
Ankle jerk: S1, 2 spinal segments

6. Identify lateral semicircular canal from the given image:

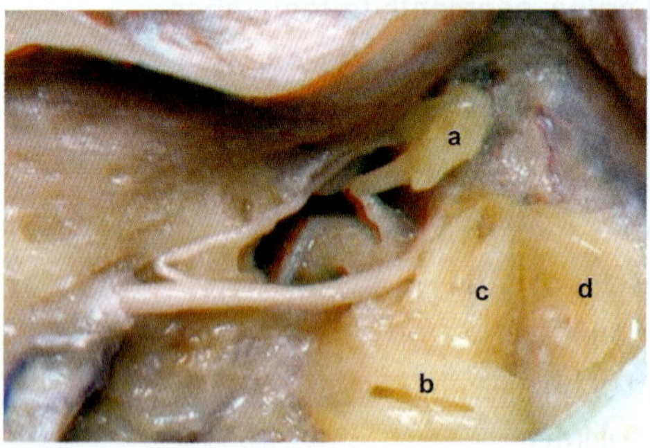

A. a B. b
C. c D. d

ANS. **C**

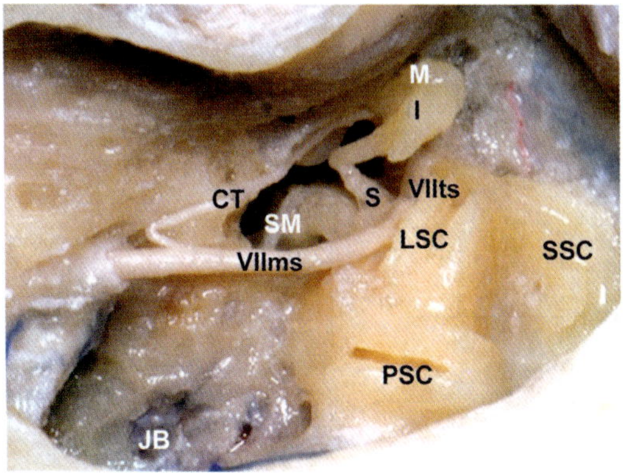

For the last few papers, operative images especially in ENT are asked. They had asked facial recess, sinus tympani. Here is a pictorial representation of these two.

Facial recess and sinus tympani relations with facial nerve and pyramidal eminence

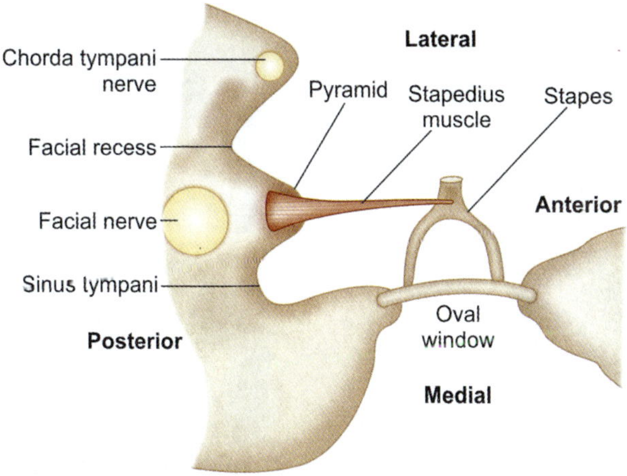

Schematic diagram showing relations of middle ear

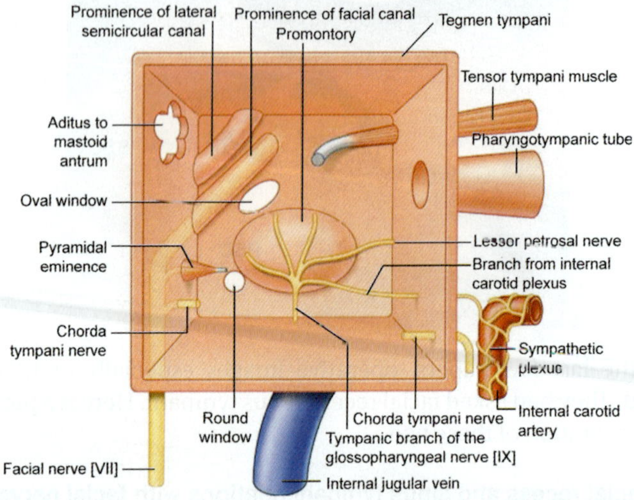

Source: Drake et al. Gray's Anatomy for students. Elsevier, www.studentconsult.com

7. Following picture exhibit which cranial nerve palsy?

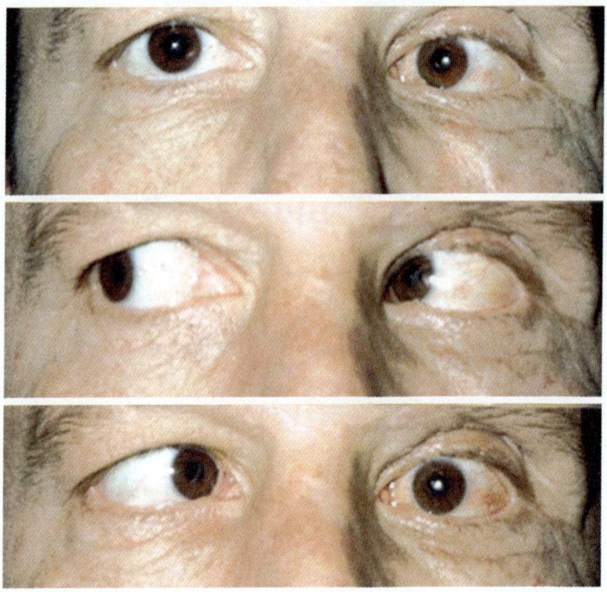

A. CN III
B. CN VI
C. CN IV
D. CN VII

ANS. **B**

This is case of abducent nerve palsy. Because right lateral gaze is normal which implies that right lateral rectus and left medial rectus are normal and also PPRF and MLF is normal. But on left gaze, adduction is normal (right medial rectus is normal), but abduction is impaired (left lateral rectus palsy).

Another important topic is extraocular muscles and their function

Functions of extraocular muscles		
Muscle	*Nerve supply*	*Action*
Superior rectus	Oculomotor (Superior division)	Elevation, adduction, intorsion
Inferior rectus	Oculomotor (Inferior division)	Depression, adduction, extortion oculomotor (Superior division)
Medial rectus	Oculomotor (Inferior division)	Abduction
Lateral rectus	Abducent	Abduction
Superior oblique	Trochlear	Depression, abduction, intorsion
Inferior oblique	Oculomotor (Inferior division)	Elevation, abduction, extortion

- All superiors are intorters
- All inferiors are extorters
- As you know is not needed **(nerve supply—LR6-SO4-O3)**
  - Lateral rectus supplied by abducens nerve
  - Superior oblique supplied by trochlear nerve
  - Rest all supplied by oculomotor nerve.

Shown below is a simple diagram demonstrating gaze mechanism and lesions at various levels.

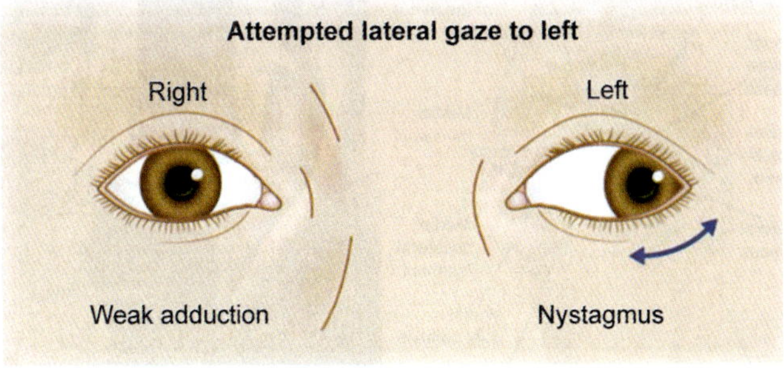

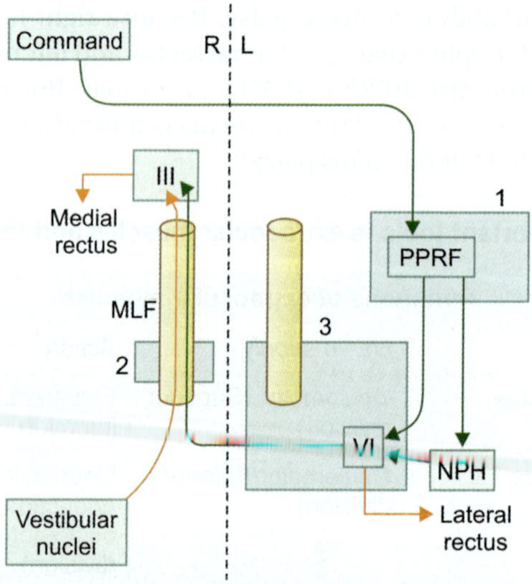

Abbreviations: NPH, nucleus prepositus hypoglossi; MLF, medial longitudinal fasciculus; PPRF, paramedian pontine reticular formation

- Lesion 1: Left horizontal gaze paresis
- Lesion 2: Right internuclear ophthalmoplegia
- Lesion 3: One and a half syndrome (Left gaze palsy along with left internuclear ophthalmoplegia).

8. Which of the following statement is not true about posterior cruciate ligament (PCL)?

A. Prevents posterior displacement of tibia on femur
B. Extrasynovial
C. Attached to anterolateral aspect of medial condyle
D. Primary action is to prevent internal rotation of knee joint

ANS. **D**

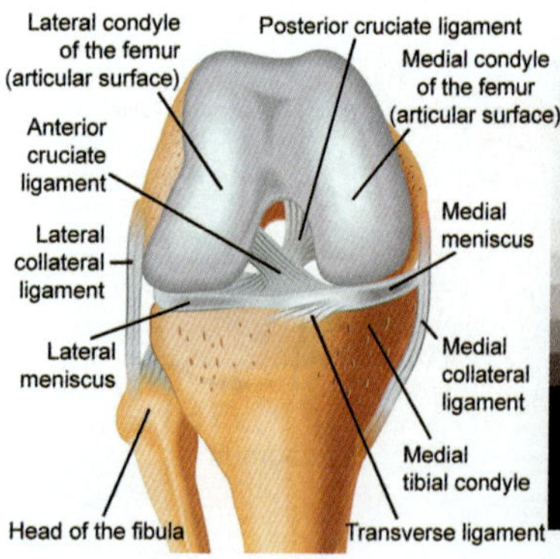

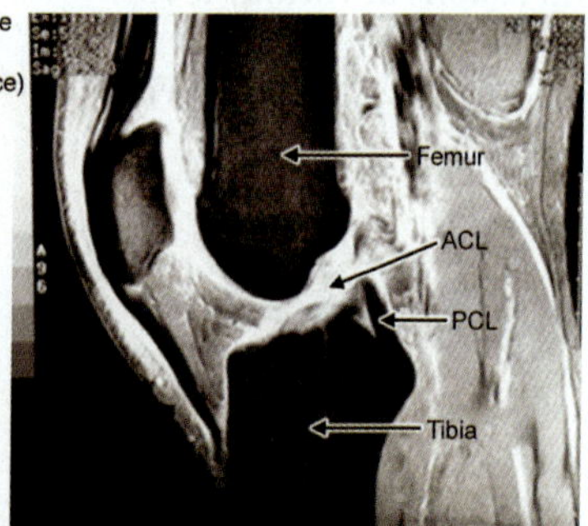

Posterior cruciate ligament

Intracapsular, extrasynovial ligament which prevent posterior displacement of tibia on femur

- PCL runs upwards, forwards and medially
- Prevent posterior dislocation of tibia on femur
- Another potential area is tests performed for ligaments of knee
- Most sensitive test for ACL and PCL: Lachman test
- Most specific test for ACL and PCL: Pivot shift test
- Best clinical test for meniscus injury: Joint line tenderness
- Investigation of choice for meniscal injury: MRI
- Gold standard investigation for meniscal injury: Arthroscopy.

Arthroscopy is a potential question especially the port size and angulation.

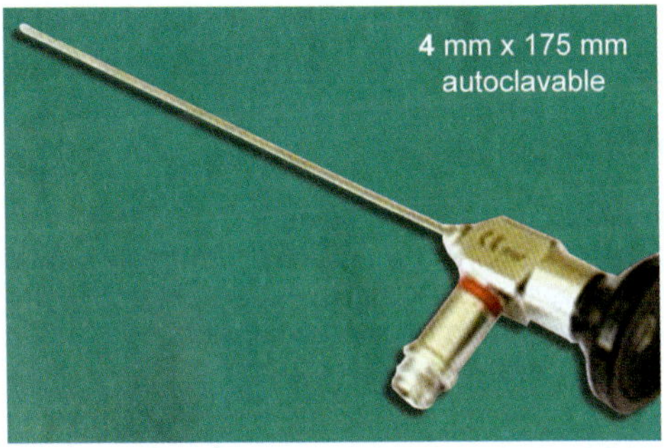

This is an arthroscope 4 mm and 30°

9. Structure passing through central tendon of diaphragm.

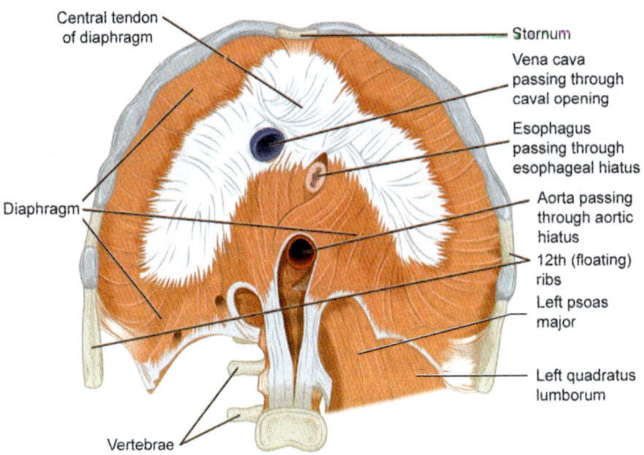

Diaphragm (inferior view)

A. Esophagus B. Aorta
C. IVC D. Sympathetic chain

ANS. **C**

Name	*Level*	*Structures passing through*
1. Aortic opening	T12 (in the median plane)	a. Aorta b. Thracic duct c. Azygos vein
2. Esophageal opening	T10 (to the left side of the median plane)	a. Esophagus b. Right and left vagus nerves c. Left gastric vessels d. Lymphatics from the lower third of the esophagus
3. Caval opening	T8 (to the right side of the median plane)	a. Inferior vena cava b. Right phrenic nerve

Development of diaphragm

- Septum transversum → Central tendon
- Pleuroperitoneal membranes → Small intermediate muscular portion
- Mesentery of esophagus → Crura
- Body wall → Peripheral muscular diaphragm
- Cervical myotomes (muscular input)

AIIMS May 2016 had given an image on development of diaphragm and asked to mark, which of these is responsible for congenital diaphragmatic hernia.

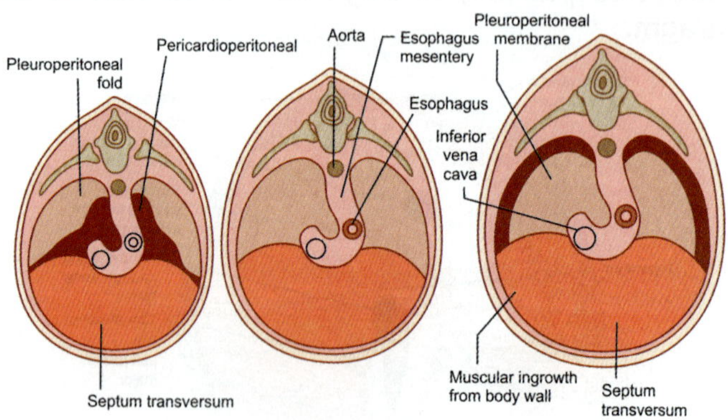

Answer to this was pleuroperitoneal membrane.

10. Which of the following sinus grows till early adulthood?

A. Maxillary
B. Ethmoid
C. Frontal
D. Sphenoid

ANS. **C**

Frontal sinus is fully developed by 18–20 years

Appearance by:	*Fully developed by:*
Maxillary sinus birth	12 years
Ethmoid sinus birth	12 years
Frontal sinus at 3 years	18–20 years
Sphenoid sinus at 8 years	12–15 years

Water's view (for maxillary sinus) Caldwell Luc view (frontal sinus)

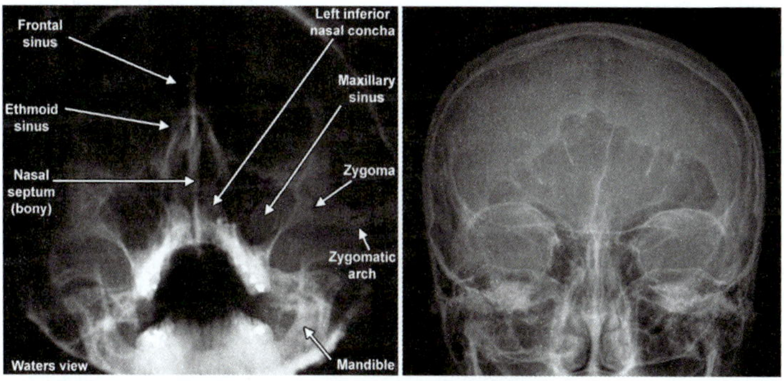

Sinus not seen in Water's view: Posterior ethmoid sinus

11. Identify the marked nerve:

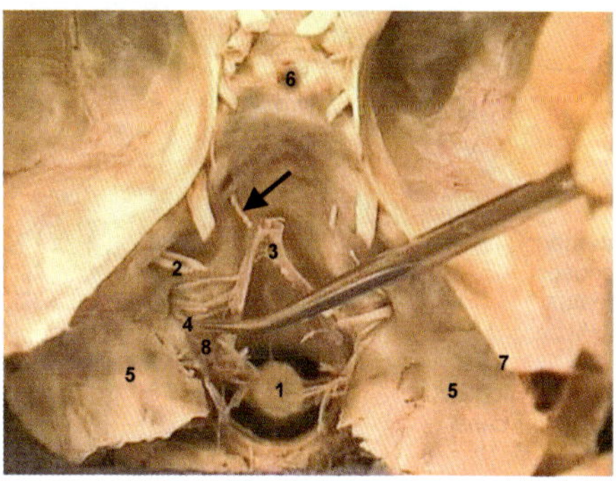

A. Abducent nerve
B. Spinal accessory nerve
C. Hypoglossal nerve
D. Labrynthine nerve

ANS. **A**

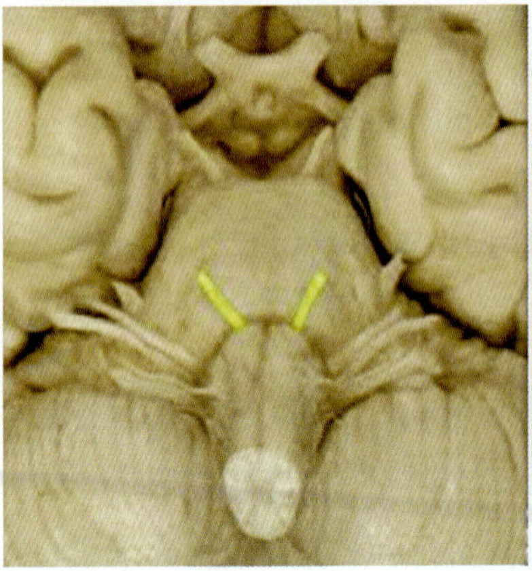

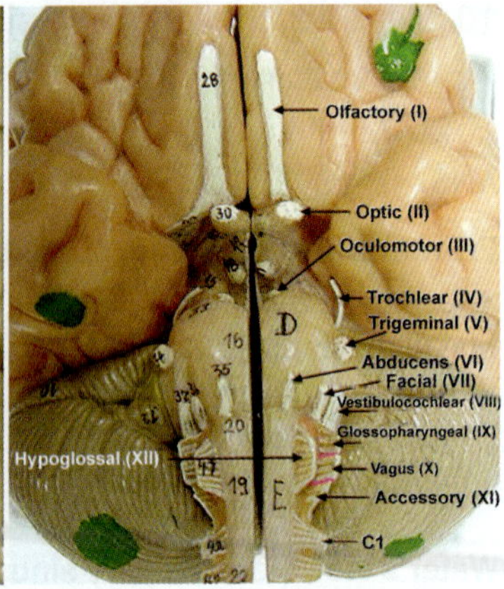

Another important topic is structures passing through the foramen of skull.

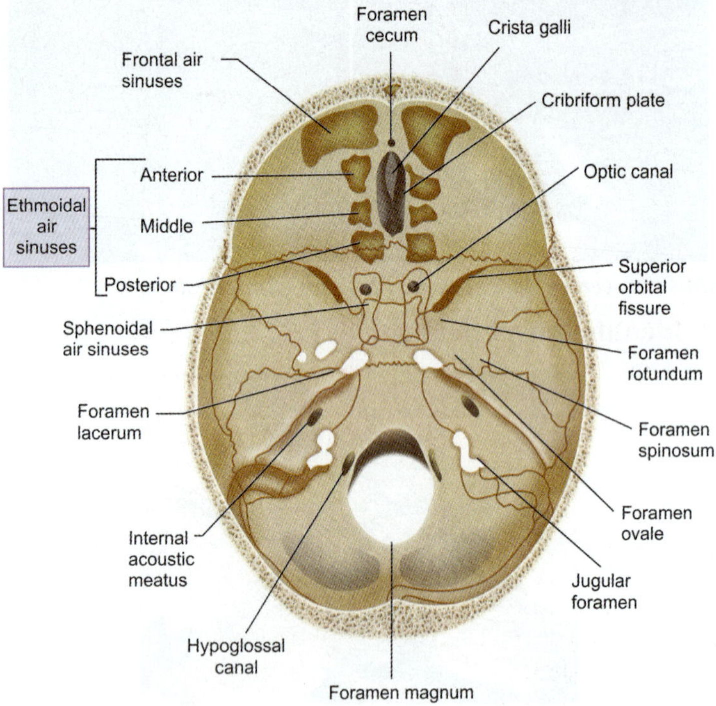

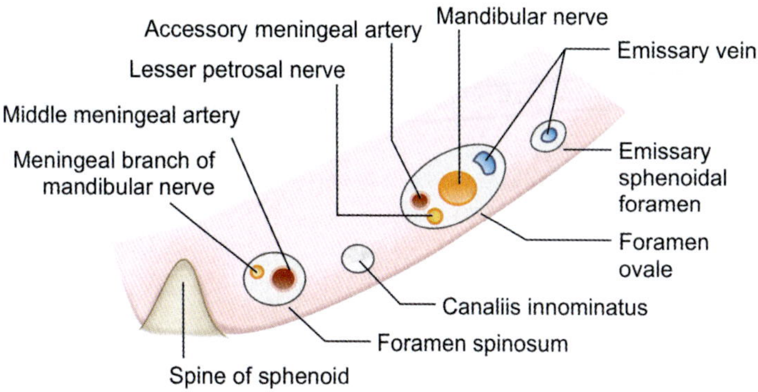

12. Holocrine cells in the given slide is:

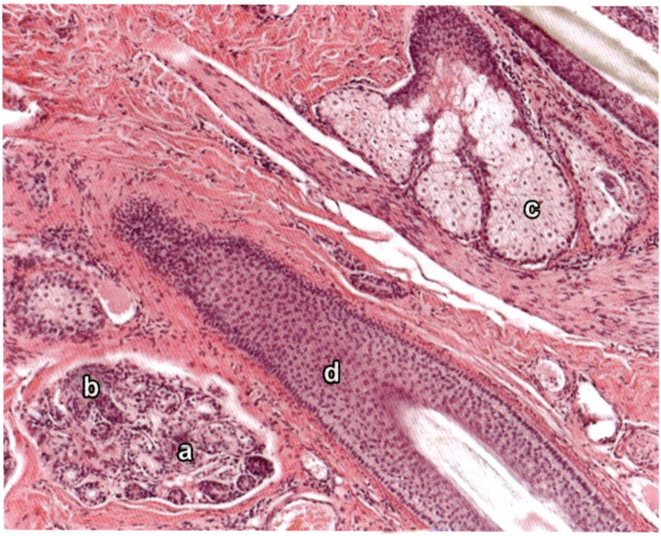

A. a B. b
C. c D. d

ANS. **C**

a: Sweat gland
b: Sweat gland duct
c: Sebaceous gland
d: Root of hair follicle
This is also a repeat from Nov 2016 paper.

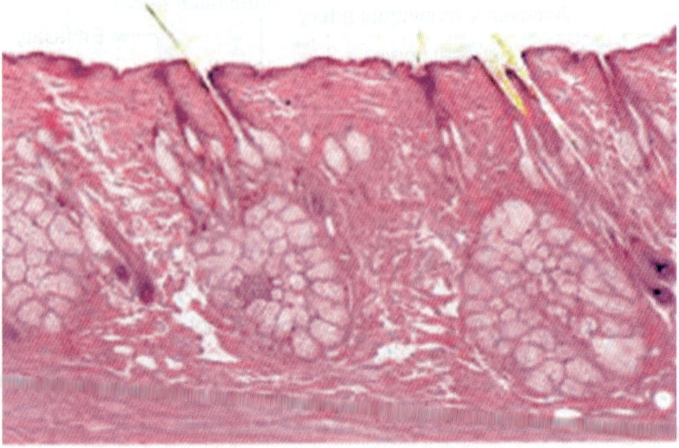

This was the image asked then and they had asked to identify the gland (Holocrine gland).

Other important glands that can be asked are:

Eccrine glands (sometimes called merocrine **glands**) are the major sweat **glands** of the human body, found in virtually all skin, with the highest density in palms and soles, then on the head, but much less on the trunk and the extremities.

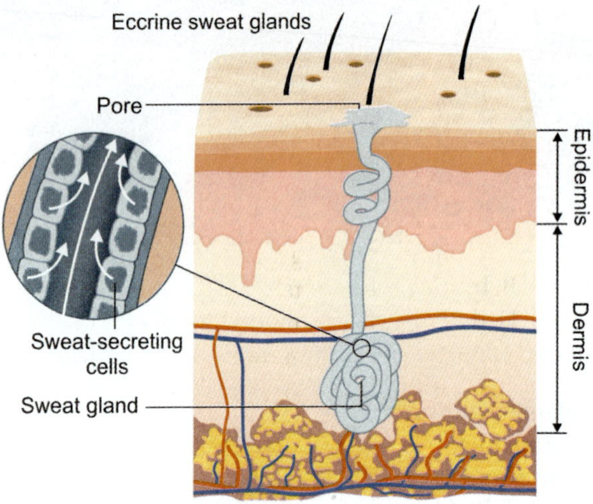

Apocrine glands in the skin and eyelid are sweat **glands**. Most **apocrine glands** in the skin are in the armpits, the groin, and the area around the nipples of the breast.

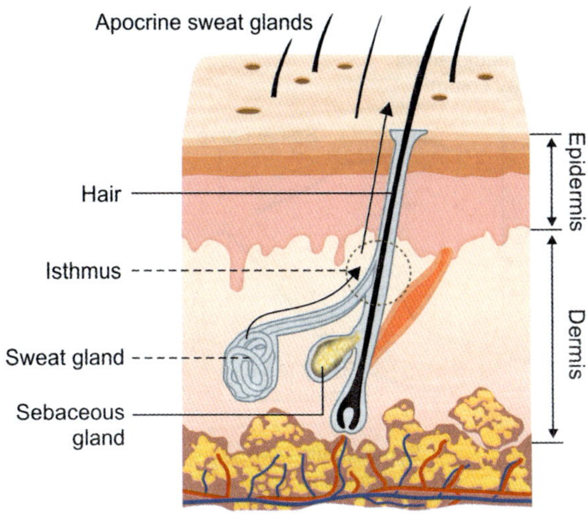

Disorders of various glands

1. Eccrine glands: Miliaria, hyperhidrosis
2. Apocrine glands: Hidradenitis, Fox-Fordyce spots
3. Sebaceous/Holocrine glands: Acne vulgaris

13. True about gray rami communicans are all *except*:

A. Unmyelinated
B. Connects to spinal nerves
C. Preganglionic
D. Present medial to white rami communicans

ANS. **C**

Each spinal nerve receives a branch called a gray rami communicans from the adjacent paravertebral ganglion of the sympathetic trunk. The gray rami communicans contain **postganglionic** nerve fibers of the sympathetic nervous system and are composed of unmyelinated nerve fibers whereas the white rami communicans are post-ganglionic and are composed of myelinated fibers.

Structure of spinal nerves: Sympathetic pathways

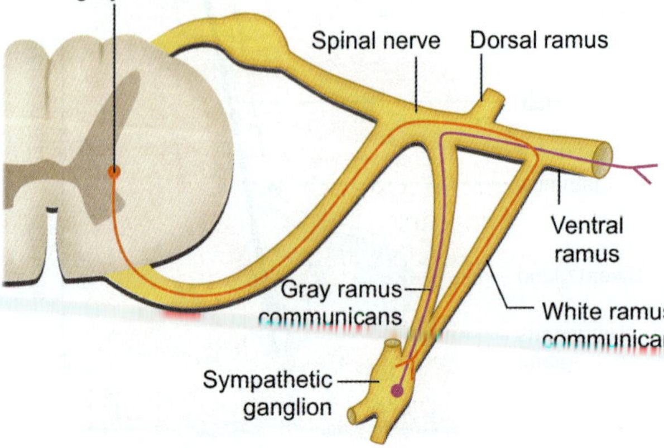

Another important topic in this portion is the Erlanger Gasser classification of nerves

Fiber types	*Function*	*Average fiber diameters (mm)*	*Average conduction velocity (m/s)*
Aα	Primary muscle spindle afferents, motor to skeletal muscle	15	100 (70–120)
Aβ	Cutaneous touch and pressure afferents	8	50 (30–70)
Aγ	Motor to muscle spindle	5	20 (15–30)
Aδ	Cutaneous temperature and pain afferents	<3	15 (12–30)
B	Sympathetic preganglionic	3	7 (3–15)
C	Cutaneous pain afferents sympathetic postganglionic	1	1 (02–2)

Numerical classification of sensory nerve fibers

Number	*Origin*	*Fiber type*
Ia	Muscle spindle, annulo-spiral ending	Aα
Ib	Golgi tendon organ	Aα
II	Muscle spindle, flower-spray ending; touch, pressure	Aβ
III	Pain and cold receptors; some touch receptors	Aδ
IV	Pain, temperature, and other receptors	Dorsal root C

14. Dense irregular collagen fibers are found in which of the following?

A. Tendon
B. Ligament
C. Dermis
D. Lamina propria

ANS. **C**

Collagen is the main structural protein in the extracellular space in the various connective tissue. Collagen consists of amino acids wound together to form triple helices to form elongated fibrils.

Dense irregular connective tissue consists of fibers that are not arranged in parallel bundles.

Dense irregular connective tissue consists of mostly collagen fibers. Fibroblasts are predominant cell type scattered sparsely across the tissue. This tissue relative to loose connective tissue contains smaller portion of ground substance.

Dense irregular connective tissue is found in:

1. Dermis of skin
2. Walls of large tubular organs
3. Organ capsules
4. Glandular tissue

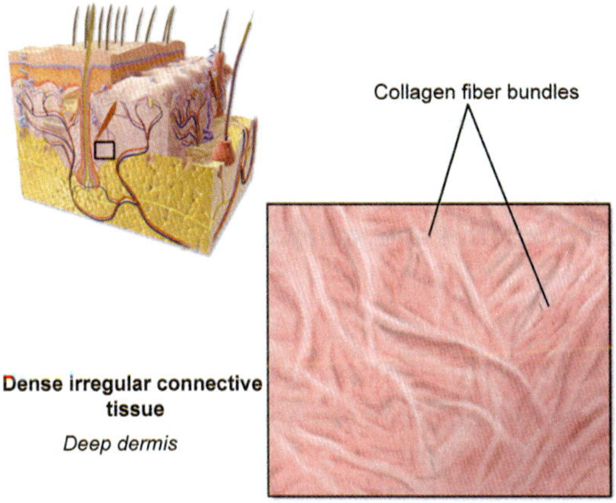

15. Injury to which of the following deep part of perineal body can lead to rectocele, cystocele and urinary incontinence?

A. Bulbospongiosus
B. Ischiocavernosus
C. Sphincter of urethra and anus
D. Pubococcygeus

ANS. **D**

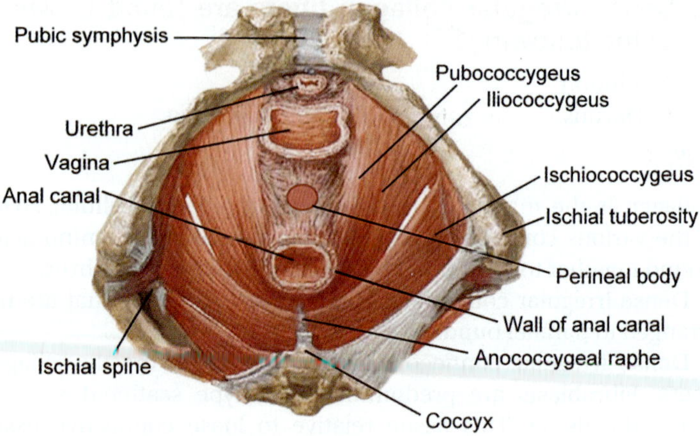

The perineal body

Structurally perineal body is an irregular fibromuscular mass, containing both collagenous and elastic fibers and both skeletal and smooth muscles.

It is the site of convergence of several muscles:

1. Bulbospongiosus
2. Superficial transverse perineal
3. Superficial part of external anal sphincter
4. Sphincter urethrae
5. Deep transverse perineal
6. Deep part of external anal sphincter
7. Levator ani

16. Which of the following is not the branch of external carotid artery in Kiesselbach plexus?

A. Anterior and posterior ethmoidal artery
B. Sphenopalatine artery
C. Greater palatine artery
D. Septal branch of superior labial artery

ANS. **A**

- Anterior and posterior ethmoidal arteries are branches of ophthalmic artery which in turn is a branch of internal carotid artery
- Sphenopalatine and greater palatine are branches of maxillary artery which in turn is a branch of external carotid artery.
- Superior labial artery is a branch of facial artery which in turn is a branch of external carotid artery.

Branches of internal carotid artery (A VIPS COMMA)

- Anterior choroidal artery
- Vidian artery
- Inferior hypophyseal artery
- Posterior communicating artery
- Superior hypophyseal artery
- Carotico tympanic artery
- Ophthalmic artery
- Middle cerebral artery
- Meningohypophyseal artery
- Anterior cerebral artery

Branch of external carotid artery

- Superior thyroid artery
- Ascending pharyngeal artery
- Lingual artery
- Facial artery
- Occipital artery
- Posterior auricular artery
- Maxillary artery
- Superficial temporal artery

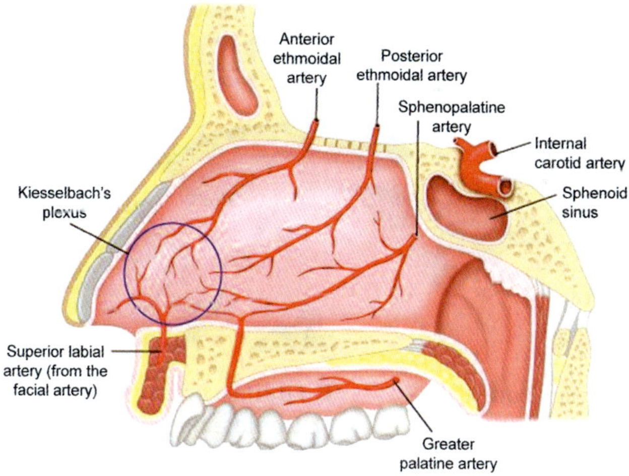

17. 1st carpal bone to ossify?

A. Scaphoid
B. Lunate
C. Capitate
D. Hamate

ANS. **C**

- Capitate: 1–3 months
- Hamate: 2–4 months
- Triquetral: 2–3 years
- Lunate: 2–4 years
- Scaphoid: 4–6 years
- Trapezium: 4–6 years
- Trapezoid: 4–6 years
- Pisiform: 8–12 years

Other important ages of ossification

1. Iliac crest: Appears by 14 years and fuses by 18 years
2. Ischial tuberosity: Appears by 16 years and fuses by 19 years
3. Coracoid process: Ossifies by 14 years
4. Acromion process: Ossifies by 17 years
5. Elbow and ankle: Fuses by 16 years
6. Humerus: Fuses by 17 years
7. Femur: Fuses by 18 years
8. Wrist and knee: Fuses by 18 years

18. Marked structure in the given image connects which of the following?

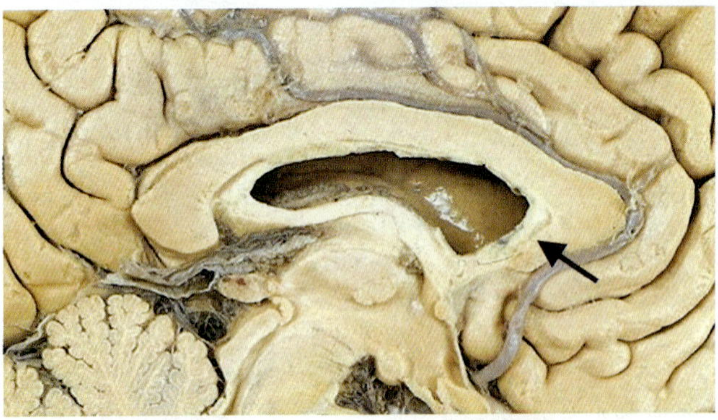

A. Striate cortex
B. Orbital cortex
C. Hippocampus
D. Dentate nucleus

ANS. **B**

Marked area is rostrum of corpus callosum

Corpus callosum is a commissural fiber which radiate into the white matter core of each hemisphere, thereafter dispersing into the cerebral cortex. Commissural fibers forming the rostrum extend laterally, below the anterior horn of the lateral ventricle, connecting the orbital surfaces of frontal lobe.

- Fibers of genu connect lateral and medial surfaces of frontal lobe
- Fibers of trunk connect neocortical areas of the hemisphere
- Fibers of splenium: Curve back into the occipital lobe.

White matter of cerebrum

1. Commissural fibers: It connects corresponding gyri of 2 hemispheres (corpus callosum and anterior commissure).
2. Association fibers: Connects one gyrus to another gyrus in same hemisphere.
3. Projection fibers: It connect cerebral cortex with lower levels in the brain and spinal cord.

Another question that can be expected is regarding agenesis of corpus callosum.

Signs of corpus callosal agenesis

Moose head appearance

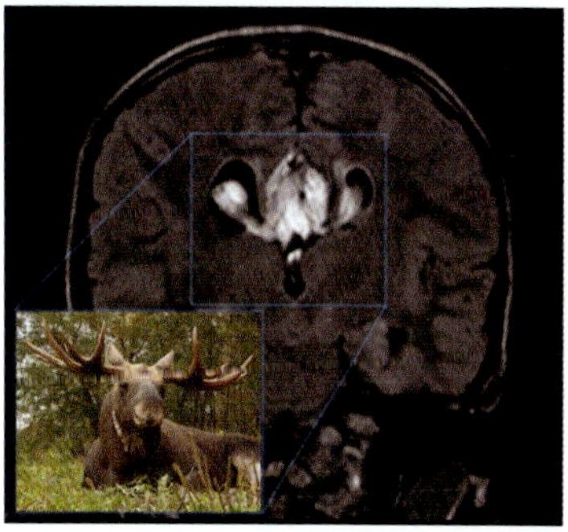

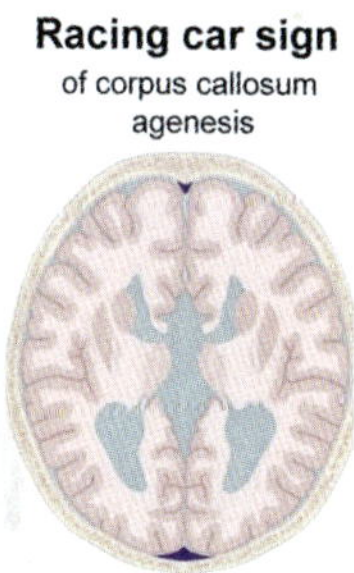

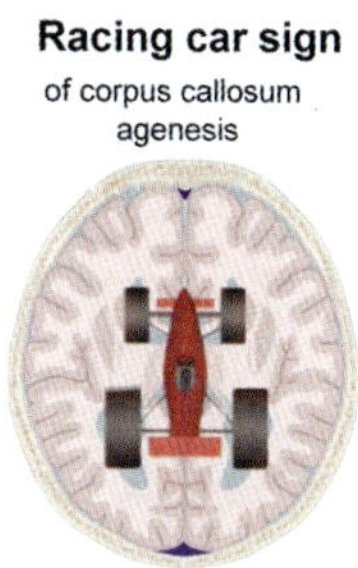

Bat wing appearance of lateral ventricle

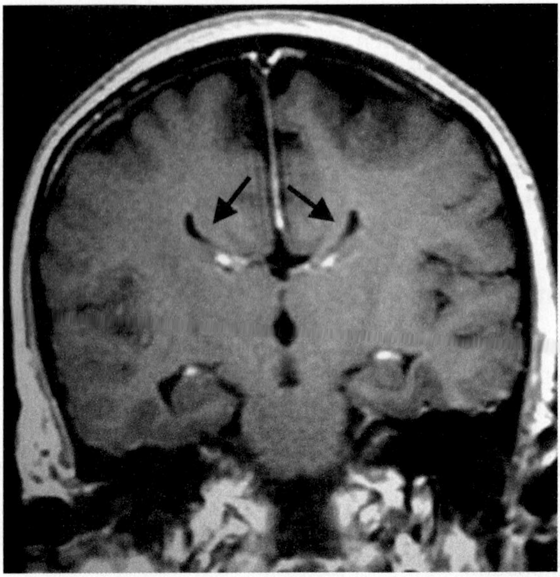

2
CHAPTER

Physiology

1. Slow waves are generated by:

A. Myentric neurons
B. Smooth muscle
C. Interstitial cells of cajal
D. Parasympathetic neurons

ANS. C

- Slow waves are the oscillating membrane potential between -60 and -40 mv in smooth muscle of GI smooth muscle.
- They are also called basal electric rhythm (BER)
- BER is maximum at duodenum (12/minute) and minimum at ileum (2/min)
- Acetyl choline increases BER and adrenergic stimulation decreases BER

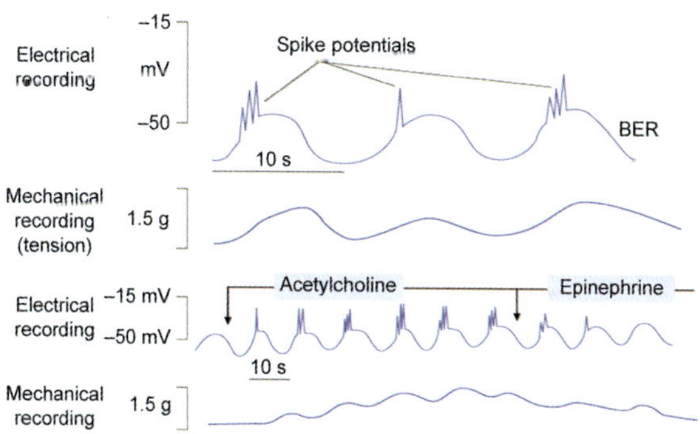

- Another topic asked in last November AIIMS 2016 was regarding migratory motor complex.
- Migratory motor complex in the gut are initiated by motilin.
- The contractions migrate at a rate of 5 cm/min and also occur at intervals of approximately 90 min.

- Migrating motor complex (MMC) appear during fasting and are inhibited by meal.
- When a meal is taken, motilin is supressed and MMC is abolished.
- Gastric secretion, bile flow and pancreatic secretion increase during each MMC.

2. Reflex responsible for tachycardia during right atrial distension is:

A. Bezold Jarisch reflex B. Bain-bridge reflex
C. Cushing reflex D. J reflex

ANS. **B**

The **Bain-bridge reflex**, also called the atrial **reflex**, is an increase in heart rate due to an increase in central venous pressure. Increased blood volume is detected by stretch receptors (cardiac receptors) located in both atria at the venoatrial junctions.

- *Stimulus:* Increase in venous return
- *Receptors:* Both right and left atria
- *Afferent:* Vagus
- *Efferent:* Sympathetic nerves
- *Effect:* Tachycardia

Other important cardiac reflexes are:

- **Bezold-Jarisch reflex:**
  - *Stimulus:* Intracardiac injection of chemicals like serotonin , capsaicin, veratridine
  - *Afferent:* Unmyelinated vagal C fibers
  - *Response:* Hypotension bradycardia
  - Mediated by serotonin
- **Marey's law**: HR and BP are inversely related.

3. Identify the stage of sleep from the given picture:

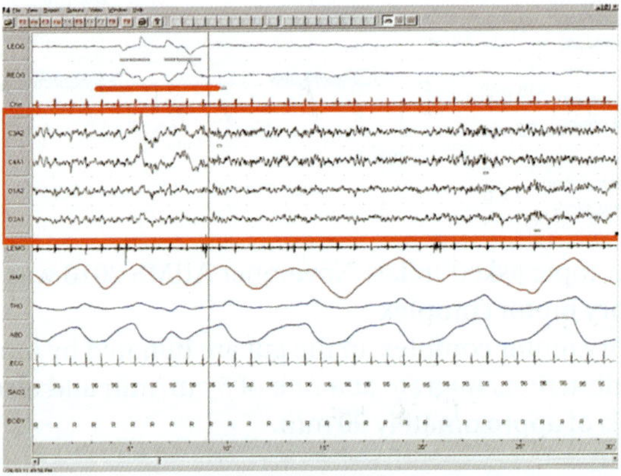

A. Stage I NREM
B. Stage 2 NREM
C. Stage 3 NREM
D. REM

ANS. **D**

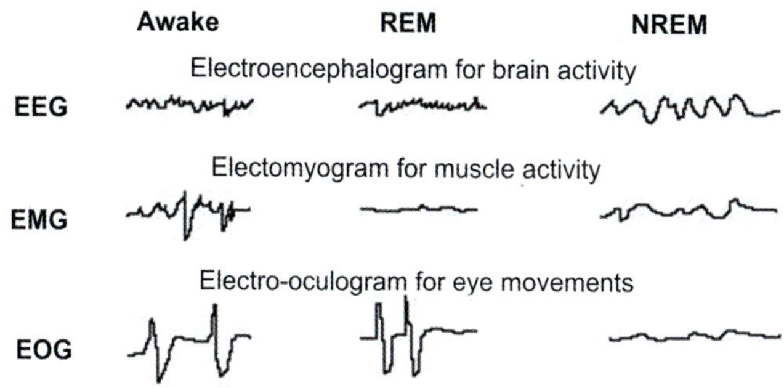

Patterns of EEG in various stages of sleep

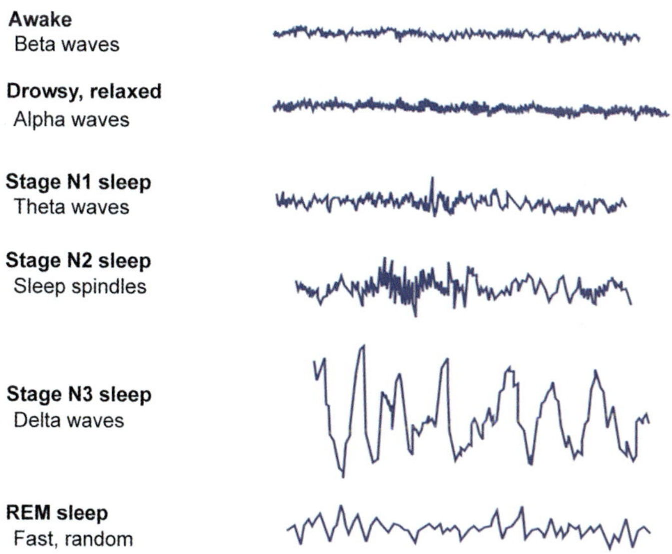

Disorders of sleep:

REM phase:

- Nightmares
- Narcolepsy
- Nocturnal penile tumescence

NREM phase

- Night terrors
- Somnambulism
- Bruxism

4. Identify the hormone from the picture.

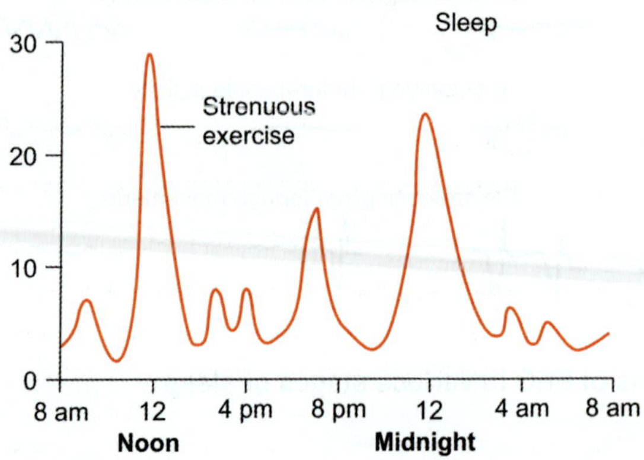

A. GH
B. Cortisol
C. Estrogen
D. Insulin

ANS. **A**

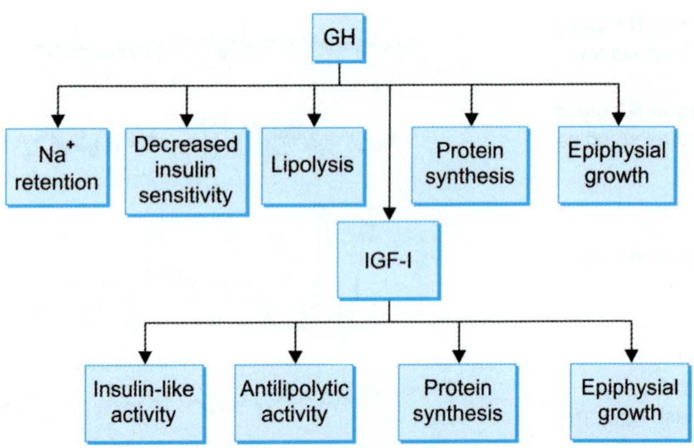

Factors that stimulate or inhibit secretion of growth hormone	
Stimulate growth hormone secretion	*Inhibit growth hormone secretion*
• Decreased blood glucose • Decreased blood free fatty acids • Starvation or fasting, protein deficiency • Trauma, stress, excitement	• Increased blood glucose • Increased blood free fatty acids • Aging • Obesity

Contd...

Contd...

• Exercise • Testosterone, estrogen • Deep sleep (stages II and IV) • Growth hormone-releasing hormone	• Growth hormone inhibitory hormone (somatostatin) • Growth hormone (exogenous) • Somatomedins (insulin-like growth factors)

5. Feed forward control system is employed during regulation of:

A. Blood volume B. pH
C. Temperature D. Blood pressure

ANS. **C**

There is a control system in our body when no stimulus is required but still the system anticipates and make corrective changes. Such system is called feed forward or anticipatory or adaptive control.

Examples

- Temperature control
- Cephalic phase of gastric secretion
- Thinking about exercise itself increases heart rate and respiratory rate.
- Role of cerebellum in motor coordination.

6. Efferent arteriolar constriction causes all *except*:

A. Decrease in GFR
B. Decrease in renal blood flow
C. Decrease in oncotic pressure in peritubular capillaries
D. Increased hydrostatic pressure in glomerular capillaries

ANS. **C**

Effect of efferent arteriolar constriction

- Efferent arteriolar constriction causes a biphasic response on GFR.
  - If there is more than three-fold increase in resistance—GFR decreases because of decrease in renal blood flow and increased colloid osmotic pressure.
  - If there is less than three-fold increase in resistance—GFR increases because of increase in pressure gradient.
- Efferent arteriolar constriction reduces peritubular capillary hydrostatic pressure, which increases net tubular reabsorption
  - Increase in proteins that escape filtration in glomerular capillaries rises oncotic pressure in the glomerular capillaries and peritubular capillaries.

Effect of afferent arteriolar constriction on GFR

There is decrease in GFR and decreased renal blood flow

Effect of dilatation of afferent arteriole on GFR

There is increase in GFR and increase in renal blood flow

Effect of dilatation of efferent arteriole on GFR (effect of ACEI on GFR)

There is decrease in GFR an increase in renal blood flow.

7. Difference in trajectory between inspiratory loop and expiratory loop in the curve is due to:

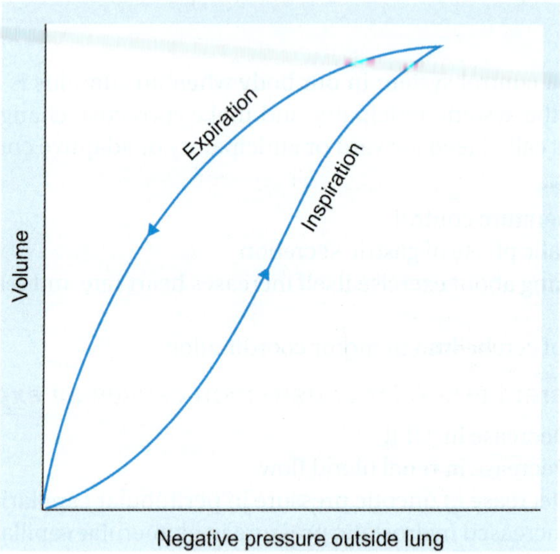

A. Difference in alveolar pressure during inspiration and expiration

B. Difference in concentration of surfactant during inspiration and expiration

C. Difference in airway resistance during inspiration and expiration

D. Inspiration is active and expiration is passive

ANS. **B**

The difference between the inspiratory and expiratory paths-hysteresis—exists because a greater transpulmonary pressure is required to open a previously closed airway, owing to a deficit of surfactant at the air-water interface, than to keep an open airway from closing, reflecting abundant surfactant.

Other important areas in respiratory physiology includes:

Spirometry

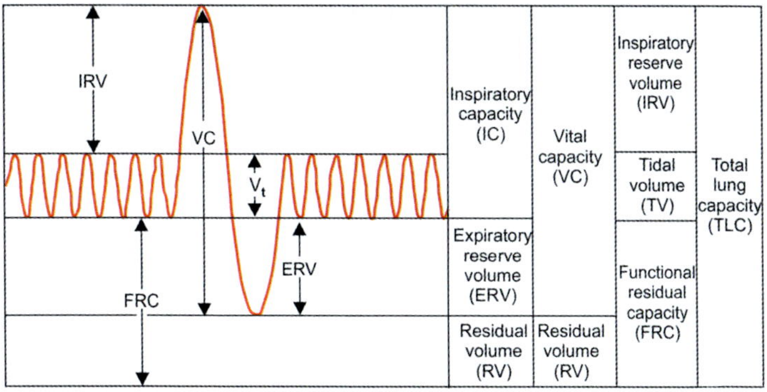

Flow volume loop in various conditions

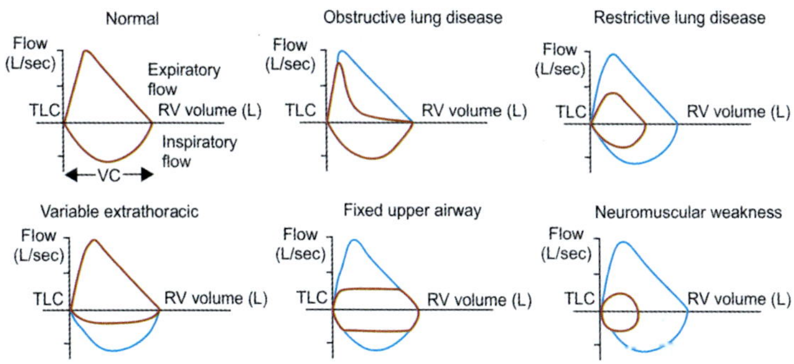

Compliance

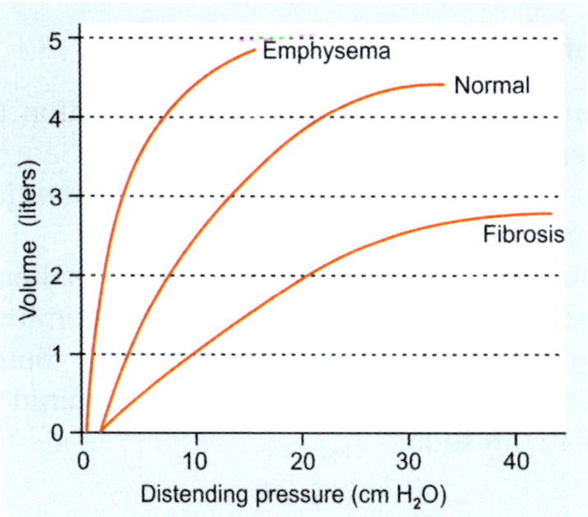

8. Absolute refractory period is due to:

A. Opening of calcium channels
B. Closure of potassium channels
C. Closure of active gates of sodium channel
D. Closure of inactive gates of sodium channel

ANS. **D**

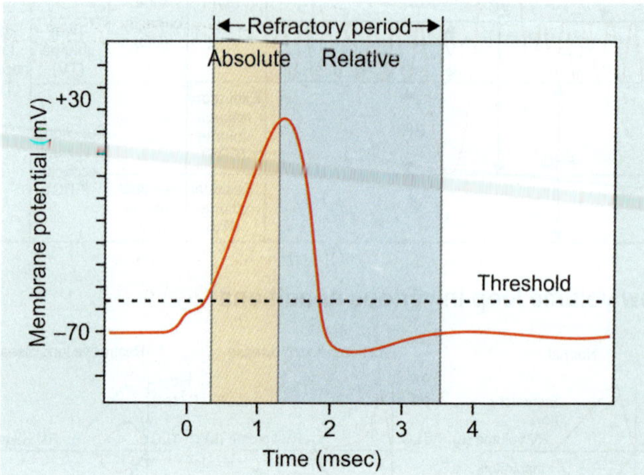

Absolute refractory period

- Corresponds to the period from the time the firing level is reached until repolarization is about one-third complete.
- There is no excitation of the nerve during this period.
- The reason for absolute refractory period is because of closure of inactivation Na^+ channels.

Relative refractory period

- Begins from the remaining part of repolarization to the end of action potential.
- Suprathreshold stimulus produces action potential in relative refractory period.
- The reason for relative refractory period is because the K^+ conductance is higher than at rest, and the membrane potential is closer to the K^+ equilibrium potential and, therefore, farther from threshold, more inward current is required to bring the membrane to threshold.

9. X,Y and Z are three ions permeable. X=-50, Y=-30. If at RMP when there is no net electrogenic transfer, what is the value of Z?

A. +20 B. –20
C. +80 D. –80

ANS. **C**

- No net electrogenic transfer at RMP means X + Y + Z = 0
- Other important points in relation to permeablity:

Nernst equation

It is used to calculate the potential generated due to movement of freely diffusible ions acrosss a semi-permeable membrane.

$$V_m = RT/zF\,(\text{In}\ c_o/c_i)$$

Where, V_m = membrane potential
R = the gas constant, 8.3 JK–1 mol^{-1}
T = temperature, 298 K
F = Faraday's constant, 96500 C mol^{-1}
z = Valence of the ion
c_o = External concentration of ion
c_i = Internal concentration of ion.

Gibb's equation

This is used to govern the distribution of ions across a semipermeable membrane. But remember, the potential generated is always calculated by Nernst equation.

Goldman's equation

The **Goldman-Hodgkin-Katz voltage equation**, more commonly known as the **Goldman equation**, is used in cell membrane physiology to determine the reversal potential across a cell's membrane, taking into account all of the ions that are permanent through that membrane.

10. Which group of nerve fibres are least susceptible to LA?

A. A alpha B. A beta
C. B D. C

ANS. **D**

Erlanger-Gasser classification of nerves			
Fiber types	*Function*	*Average fiber diameters (μm)*	*Average conduction velocity (m/s)*
Aα	Primary muscle spindle afferents, motor to skeletal muscle	15	100 (70–120)
Aβ	Cutaneous touch and pressure afferents	8	50 (30–70)
Aγ	Motor to muscle spindle	5	20 (15–30)
Aδ	Cutaneous temperature and pain afferents	<3	15 (12–30)
B	Sympathetic preganglionic	3	7 (3–15)
C	Cutaneous pain afferents sympathetic postganglionic	1	1 (02–2)

LA susceptiblity: A delta>gamma>A beta>A alpha>B>C
Hypoxia: B > A > C
Pressure: A > B > C
[*Source:* The New York School of Regional Anesthesia (NYSORA)]

3

CHAPTER

Biochemistry

1. A 10-year-old boy rapidly develops hypoglycemia after moderate activity. Blood examination reveals raised levels of ketone bodies, lactic acid and triglyceides. On examination, liver and kidney were enlarged. Histopathology of liver shows deposits of glycogen in excess amount. Diagnosis?

A. Von Gierke's disease B. Cori's disease
C. Mcardle's disease D. Pompe's disease

ANS. **A**

Glycogen-storage diseases				
Type	*Defective enzyme*	*Organ affected*	*Glycogen in the affected organ*	*Clinical features*
I Von Gierke	Glucose-6-phosphatase	Liver and kidney	Increased amount; normal structure	Massive enlargement of the liver. Failure to thrive. Severe hypoglycemia, ketosis, hyperuricemia, hyperlipemia
II Pompe	α-1, 4-glucosidase (lysosomal)	All organs	Massive increase in amount; normal structure	Cardiorespiratory failure causes death, usually before age 2

Contd...

Contd...

III Cori	Amylo-1, 6-glucosidase (debranching enzyme)	Muscle and liver	Increased amount; short outer branches	Like type I but milder course
IV Andersen	Branching enzyme (α-1, 4 → α-1, 6)	Liver and spleen	Normal amount; very long outer branches	Progressive cirrhosis of the liver. Liver failure causes death, usually before age 2
V McArdle	Phosphorylase	Muscle	Moderately increased amount; normal structure	Limited ability to perform strenuous exercise because of painful muscle cramps. Otherwise patient is normal and well developed
VI Hers	Phosphorylase	Liver	Increased amount	Like type I, but milder course
VII	Phospho-fructokinase	Muscle	Increased amount; normal structure	Like type V
VIII	Phosphorylase kinase	Liver	Increased amount; normal structure	Mild liver enlargement. Mild hypoglycemia

Important points regarding glycogen storage disorders

- Most common glycogen storage disorder: Von gierke's disease
- Glycogen storage disorder with cardiomegaly:Pompe's
- Glycogen storage disorder with liver cirrhosis:Anderson's disease
- Burgundy colour urine after exercise:Mcardle disease
- Features same as von gierke,but kidneys not enlarged:Cori's
- Glycogen storage disorder which is also a lysosomal disorer: Pompe's disease.

2. Which a.a does not include post-translational modification?

A. Selenocysteine   B. Triiodothyronine
C. Hydroxyproline   D. Hydroxylysine

ANS. **A**

Selenocysteine—> UGA
Pyrolysine—>UAG
Both of these are examples of cotranslational modification of selenium-containing enzymes are:

- Glutathione peroxidase
- Deiodinase
- Thioredoxin reductase.

Examples of post-translational modification

- Methylation
- Acetylation
- Phosphorylation
- Ubiquitylation
- Sumoylation.

Examples of post-trancsriptional modification

- 5-Capping
- Poly A Tailing
- Splicing
- miRNA and siRNA.

3. Glucosamines used in following condition:

A. Arthritis B. Niemann-Pick disease
C. Alzheimers disease D. Cancer

ANS. **A**

Glucosamine ($C_6H_{13}NO_5$) is an amino sugar and a prominent precursor in the biochemical synthesis of glycosylated proteins and lipids. Glucosamine is part of the structure of the polysaccharides chitosan and chitin, which compose the exoskeletons of crustaceans and other arthropods, as well as the cell walls of fungi and many higher organisms.

It is produced commercially by the hydrolysis of crustacean exoskeletons or, less commonly, by fermentation of a grain such as corn or wheat.

Commonly sold forms of glucosamine are glucosamine sulfate, glucosamine hydrochloride, and *N*-acetylglucosamine. Of the three commonly available forms of glucosamine, only glucosamine sulfate is given a "likely effective" rating for treating osteoarthritis. Glucosamine is often sold in combination with other supplements such as chondroitin sulfate and methylsulfonylmethane.

Salient features about GAG (Glycosaminoglycans)

- Most abundant GAG: chondroitin sulfate
- GAG with no uronic acid: Keratin
- GAG with no sulfate group: Hyaluronic acid
- GAG not covalently bound: Hyaluronic acid
- Only intracellular GAG: Heparin

4. Which vitamin is required for glycogen phosphorylase?

A. Pyridoxal phosphate (PLP)
B. Thiamine diphosphate (TPP)
C. Riboflavin
D. Lipoic acid

ANS. **A**

Other important roles of pyridoxine

- Involved in transamination reaction
- Involved in heme synthesis
- Required for glycogenolysis
- Required for transsulfuration reaction
- For decarboxylation of amino acids:
  - Glutamate → GABA
  - 5-HIAA → serotonin
  - DOPA → Dopamine
- Pyridoxine facilitates peripheral conversion of DOPA to dopamine, hence pyridoxine is contraindicated in parkinsonism.
- Pyridoxine is used in treatment of homocystinuria and hyperoxaluria.

5. Structure of DNA is shown. What are the bonds between 2 nitrogenous bases?

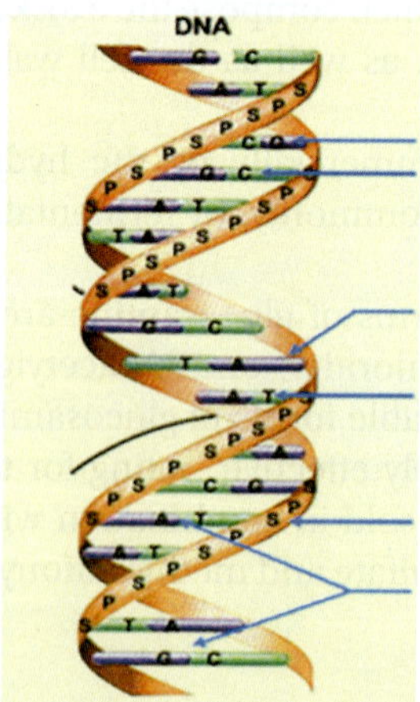

A. 3-5 phosphodiester bonds
B. 2-5 phosphodiester bonds
C. Hydrogen bonds
D. Covalent bonds

ANS. **C**

Nitrogenous Base + Pentose Sugar → Nucleoside
Nitrogenous Base + Pentose Sugar + Phosphate → Nucleotide

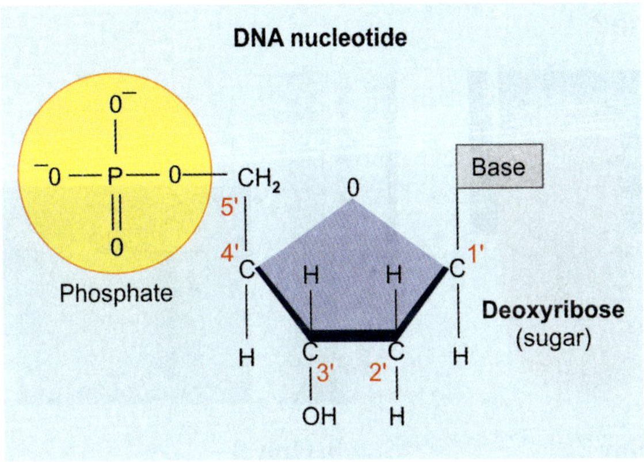

Some important points about nucleotides:

- Adenine is the only base without oxygen atom
- Mean intracellular concentration of ATP is 1 mmol/L
- Nucleotide acting as methyl group donor is: S-adenosyl methionine
- Nucleotide acting as secondary messenger: cAMP, cGMP
- Nucleotide absorb ultraviolet light close to 260 nm.
- Energy liberated by hydrolysis of each of the terminal phosphoryl group is about 7 kcal/mol.

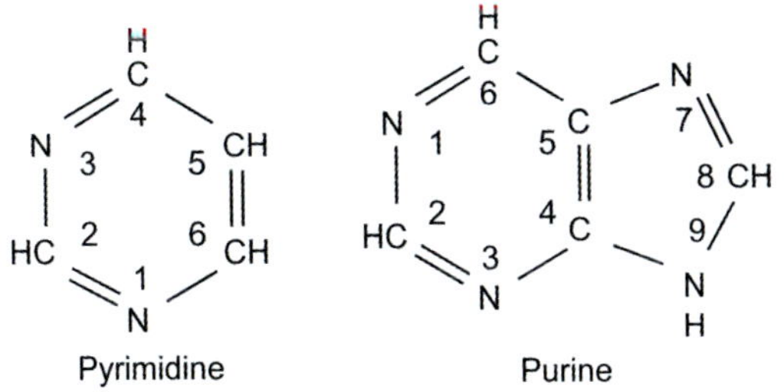

Purine ring:

- Glycine C4 C5 N7
- Aspartate N1
- Glutamine N3 N9

- Tetrahydrofolate-C2 C8
- Carbon dioxide-C6.

Pyrimidine

- Glutamine-N3
- Aspartic acid-C4 C5 C6 N1
- CO_2 provides C2.

6. Following are the tests done for patients, sugar and ketones which will be positive in starvation state in urine?

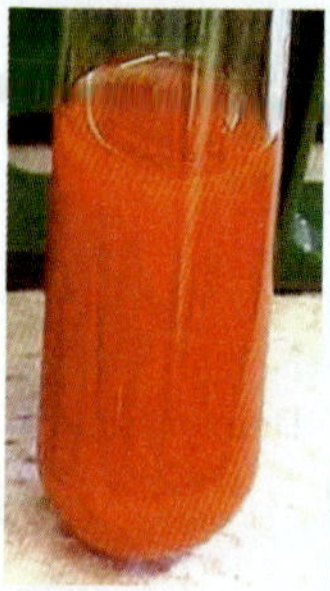
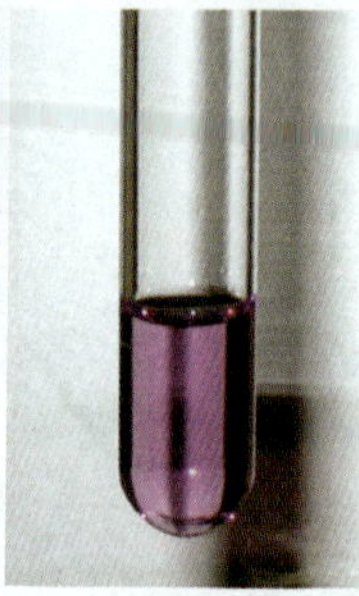
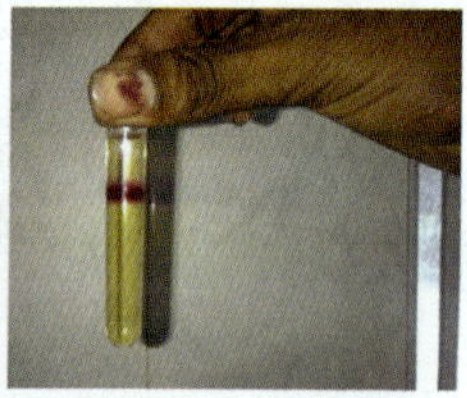

A. Only 2
B. Only 3
C. 1 and 2
D. 2 and 3

ANS. **B**

- First image shows positive Benedict's test.
- Second image shows positive biuret test
- Third image shows positive Rothera's test
- In prolonged starvation, ketone bodies are accumulated.

	I	*II*	*III*	*IV*	*V*
	0–4 hours	*4–16 hours*	*16–32 hours*	*32 hours to 24 days*	*24 days and on*
Origin of blood glucose	Exoge-nous	Glycogen, hepatic GNG	Hepatic GNG, glycogen	Hepatic and renal GNG	Hepatic and renal GNG
Tissues using glucose	All	All except liver Muscle and adipose tissue of diminished rate	All except liver Muscle and fat tissue at rates inter-mediary between II and IV	Brain, red blood cells, renal medulla. Small amount by muscle	Brain at a diminished rate, red blood cells, renal medulla

Contd...

Contd...

Major fuel of brain	Glucose	Glucose	Glucose	Glucose, ketone bodies	Ketone bodies, glucose

Salient features about starvation

- First substrate metabolized in starvation is glycogen (up to 12–18 hours)
- Once glycogen stores are completely used up, gluconeogenesis begins.
- For converting 1 mol of glucose, 6 ATP is utilized.
- Liver and RBC does not use ketone body during starvation
- Brain does not use fatty acid.
- Retina completely depend on glucose as fuel for energy.

7. Which is not involved in iron metabolism?

A. Transthyretin B. Ceruloplasmin
C. Hepcidin D. Ferritin

ANS. **A**

Ceruloplasmin is a Cu^{+} containing enzyme for ferroxidase activity (Fe^{2+} – > Fe^{3+})

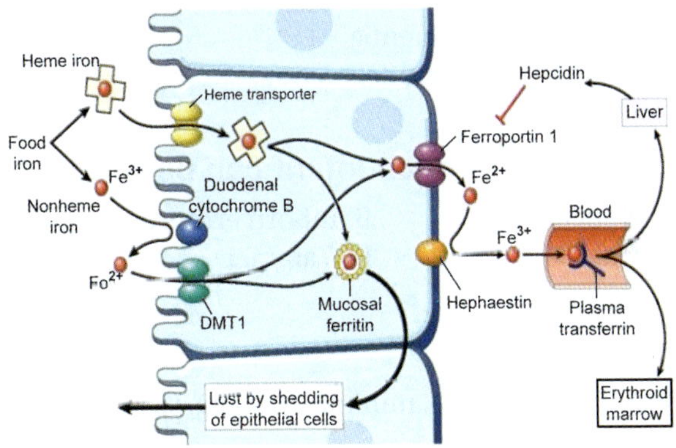

Duodenal epithelial cell uptake of heme and nonheme iron

- Acute phase proteins
- Positive:
  - C-reactive protein
  - Ceruloplasmin
  - Haptoglobin

Negative acute phase protein:

- Transferrin
- Albumin

- Transthyretin
- Retinol binding protein.

8. In severe combined immunodeficiency (SCID), what type of DNA repair is defective?

A. Double strand break repair
B. Nucleotide excision repair
C. End joining repair (NHEJ)
D. Homologous end joining

ANS. **C**

DNA repair mechanisms and disorders associated with it:

- Nucleotide excision repair (Xenoderma pigmentosa)
- Mismatch repair (HNPCC)

Recombinant repair:

- Ataxia telangiectasia
- Fanconi's syndrome
- Bloom's syndrome.

Disorders of T and B cell

T cell:

- DiGeorge syndrome
- SCID

B cell:

- X-linked agammaglobulinemia
- Common variable immunodeficiency
- IgA deficiency.

9. Dried blood drop of an infant can be used to know:

A. Blood sugar
B. Inborn errors of metabolism
C. Hepatitis
D. Cataract

ANS. **B**

Dried blood drop test:

Advantage: Minimal volume, minimal training, ease of transport.
Used for:

- Phenylketonuria (PKU)
- Galactosemia
- Maple syrup urine disease (MSUD)
- Sickle cell disease.

Inborn errors of amino acid metabolism associated with peculiar odor	
Inborn error in metabolism	*Urine odor*
Glutaric acidemia (Type II)	Sweaty feet, acrid
Isovaleric acidemia	Sweaty feet, acrid
Maple syrup urine disease	Maple syrup
Hypermethioninemia	Boiled cabbage
Multiple carboxylase deficiency	Tomcat urine
Phenylketonuria	Mousy or musty
Trimethylaminuria	Rotting fish
Tyrosinemia	Boiled cabbage, rancid butter

Rate limiting enzymes in metabolic pathways

- Glycolysis—Phosphofructokinase 1
- Citric acid/TCA cycle—Isocitrate dehydrogenase
- Bile acid synthesis—7 alpha dehydroxylase
- Cholesterol synthesis—HMG CoA reductase
- Ketone body synthesis—HMG CoA synthase
- Fatty acid synthesis—Acetyl CoA carboxylase
- Fatty acid oxidation—Carnitine palmitoyltransferase 1
- Urea cycle—Carbamoyl phosphate synthase 1
- Pyrimidine synthesis—Carbamoyl phosphate synthetase 2
- Purine synthesis—PRPP glutamyl amidotransferase
- Heme synthesis—ALA synthase
- Testosterone synthesis—Cholesterol desmolase
- Catecholamine synthesis—Tyrosine hydroxylase

4
CHAPTER

Pathology

1. Storage period of 35 days for blood is seen with:

A. Citrate-phosphate-dextrose (CPD)
B. Citrate-phosphate-dextrose-alanine-1 (CPDA-1)
C. Acid-citrate-dextrose (ACD)
D. Citrate-phosphate-dextrose-dextrose (CP2D)

ANS. **B**

Storage period and preservatives

- CPD—21 days
- ACD—21 days
- CPDA—35 days
- SAGM—42 days

SAGM: Saline, adenine, glucose, mannitol
Function of SAGM: Increases shelf life of red blood cell (RBC)

CPD:

- Citrate—Ca^{2+} chelator
- Phosphate—increased 2, 3, DPG and buffering
- Dextrose—nutrition.

2. When you add calcium and thromboplastin to platelet poor plasma, which pathway is assessed:

A. Extrinsic
B. Intrinsic
C. Fibrinolysis
D. Common

ANS. **A**

- Thrombin time: Reflects conversion of fibrinogen to fibrin
- Prothrombin time: Reflects extrinsic pathway of platelet poor plasma + tissue factor + calcium replaces platelet phospholipid

- Activated partial thromboplastin time (APTT): Measures intrinsic and common pathway.
- Platelet poor plasma + surface activator (kaolin, silica, etc.) + phospholipid + calcium

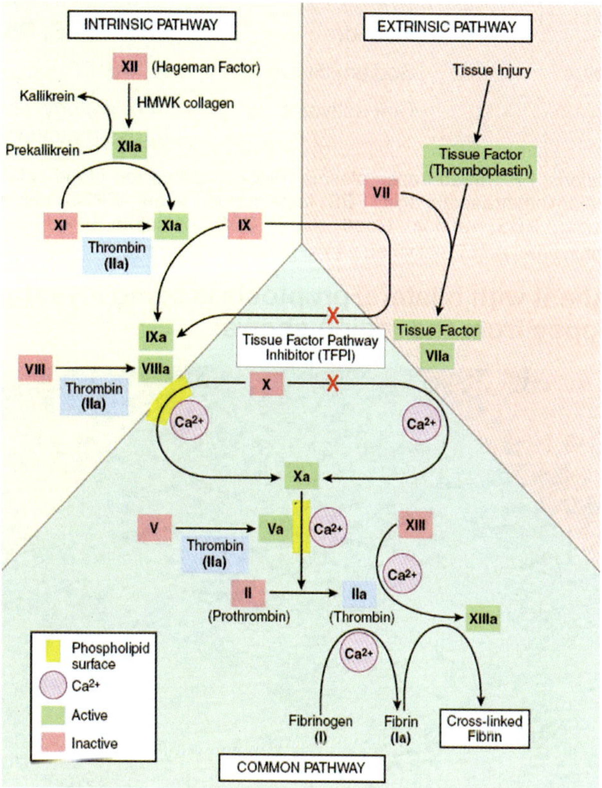

3. Which anticoagulant is used for electrolyte estimation?

A. Ethylenediaminetetraacetic acid (EDTA)
B. Citrate
C. Sodium fluoride (NaF)
D. Lithium heparin

ANS. **D**

Component	*Temperature*	*Can be used up to*
Platelet	20–24 degrees	5 days
FFP	–30 degrees	1 year
Whole blood	20–24 degrees	1 day
PRBC	0–4 degrees	42 days

Contd...

Contd...

Color	*Anticoagulant*	*Use*
Violet	EDTA	CBC, hemogram
Green	Heparin	Serum electrolytes
Gray	Fluoride	FBS, PPBS, RBS
Light blue	Sodium citrate	PT, APTT
Red	Clot activator	Immunology, serology (cross matching)

Abbreviations: FFP, fresh-frozen plasma; PRBC, packed red blood cells; EDTA, ethylenediaminetetraacetic acid; FBS, fasting blood sugar; PPBS, post-prandial blood sugar, RBS, random blood sugar; CBC, complete blood count; PT, prothrombin time; APTT, activated partial prothrombin time

4. Patient with bilateral proptosis is being investigated. Biopsy from the region shows:

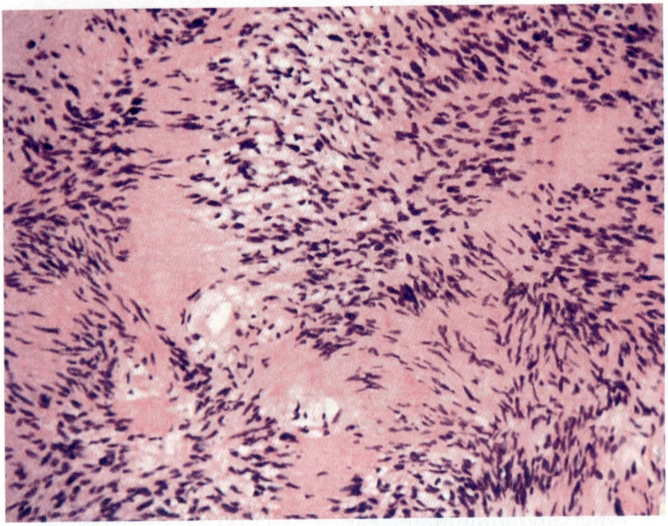

A. Leiomyoma
B. Schwannoma
C. Rhabdomyosarcoma
D. Fibromatosis

ANS. **B**

- Schwannoma is a favorite topic for AIIMS. Previously had asked to mark Antoni A and B, Verocay bodies

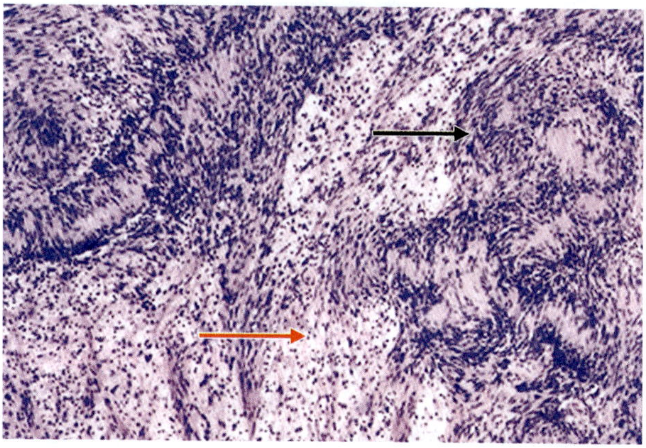

- Dense area is Antoni A (black arrow) and less dense area is Antoni B (red arrow)
- Other important histological slides of brain malignancies they can ask are:

Meningioma (whorled pattern and psammoma bodies)

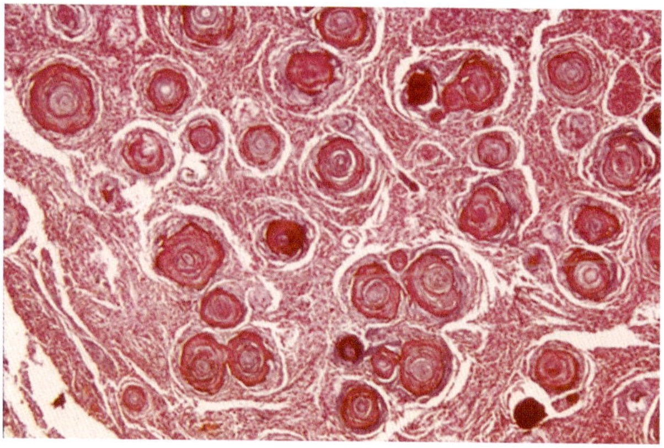

Medulloblastoma (small round blue cell tumor)

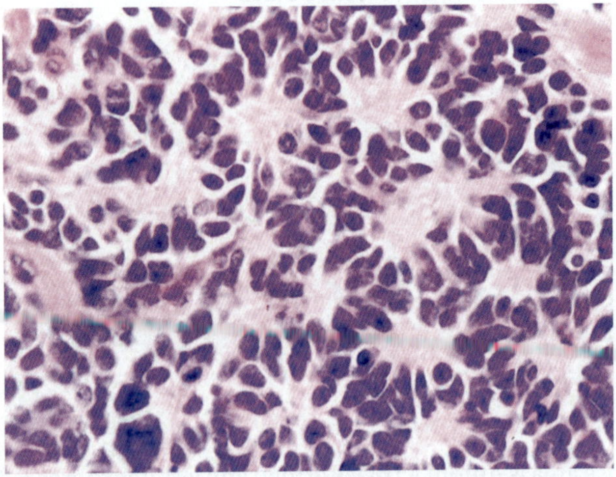

Ependymoma (characteristic perivascular pseudorosette)

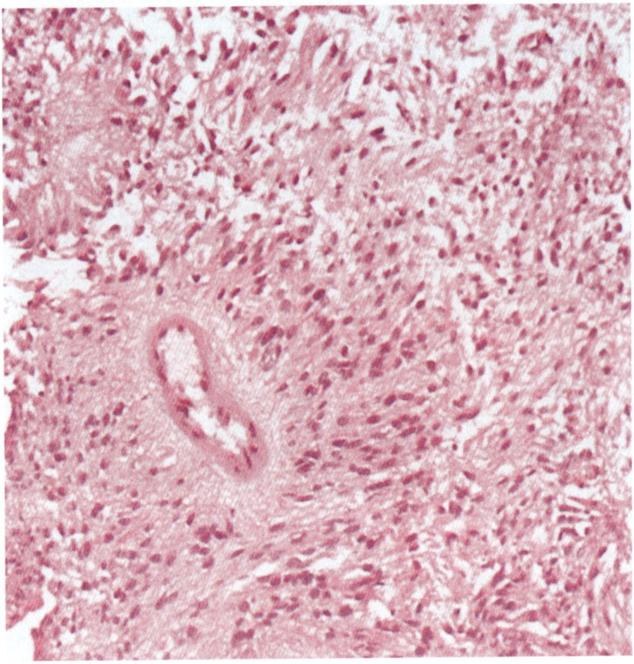

Glioblastoma multiformes (densely cellular tumor with necrosis and pseudopalisading of tumor cell nuclei)

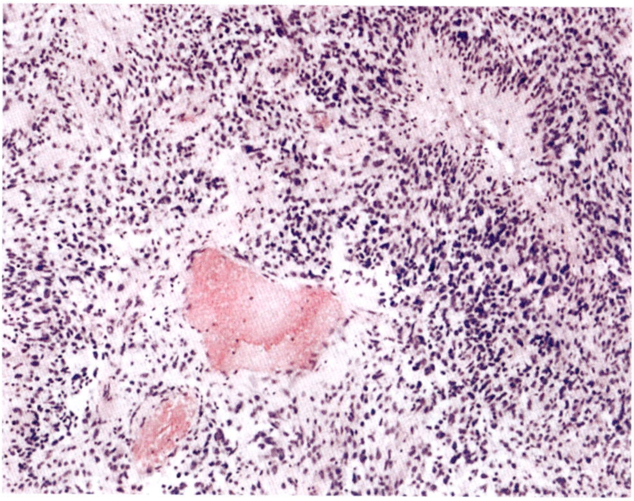

Pilocytic astrocytoma (rosenthal fibers)

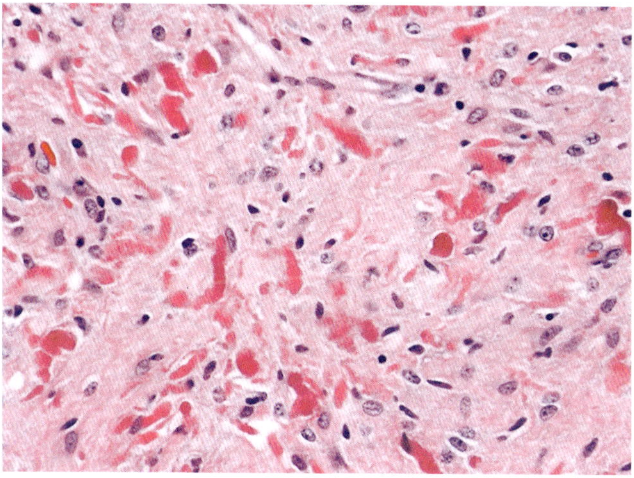

5. Patient with hemoglobin A (HbA) 2–3% add fetal hemoglobin (HbF) 97%, patient smear will have:

1.

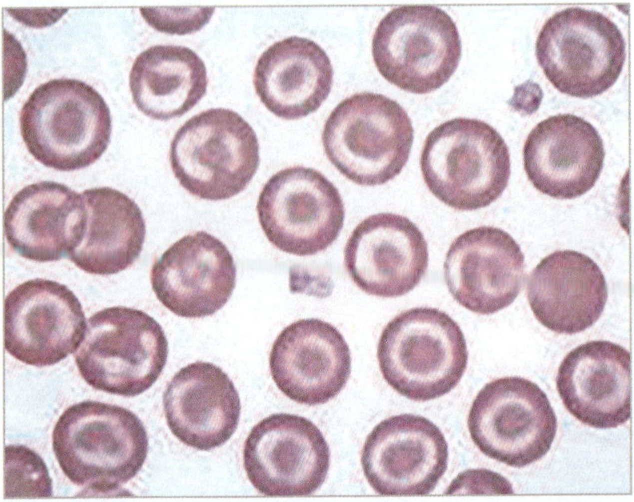

2.

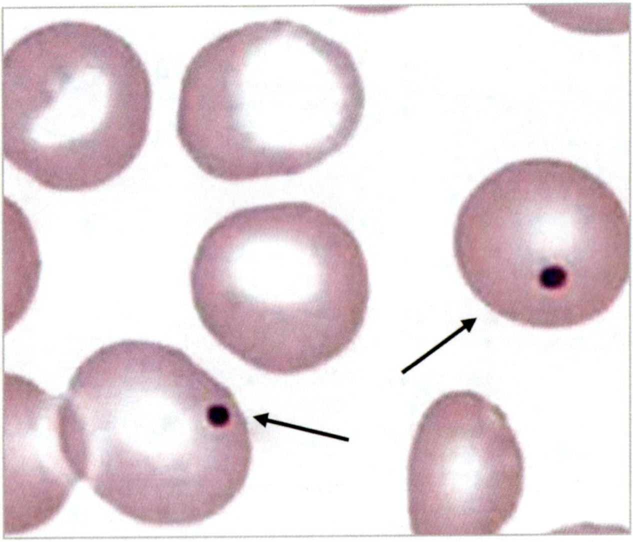

3.

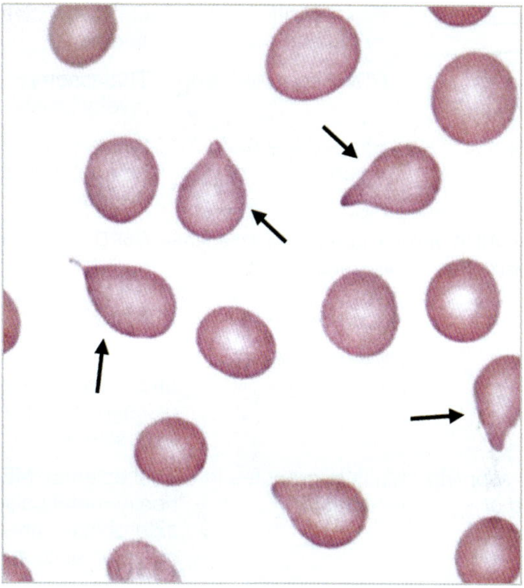

A. 1 and 2
B. 1 and 3
C. 1 and 4
D. 1, 2 and 3

ANS. **D**

Findings in thalassemia major

- Target cells
- Howell-Jolly (HJ) bodies
- Tear drop cells/dacryocytes
- Nucleated RBCs
- Anisopoikilocytosis

Shape	*Appearance*	*Causes*
Spherocyte	No central pallor	Hereditary spherocytosis, AIHA, G6PD deficiency anemia
Acanthocyte	Irregular spicules on their surfaces	Abetalipoproteinemia
Elliptocytosis	Elliptical shape	Hereditary elliptocytosis
Echinocyte (burr cell)	Undulation on surface	Uremia and anemia of CRF
Schistocyte (helmet cell)	Irregular shape	Microangiopathic hemolytic anemia (MAHA)

Contd...

Contd...

Bite cell	Pinched off cytoplasm	G6PD deficiency anemia
Tear drop cells (dacryocytes)	RBC like a tear drop	Thalassemia, myelofibrosis
Sickle cells	Shaped like half moon	Sickle cell anemia, hemoglobin sickle cell disease

Abbreviations: AIHA, autoimmune hemolytic anemia; G6PD, glucose-6 phosphate dehydrogenase; CRF, chronic renal failure

Name/contents	*Appearance*	*Conditions*
Target cells	Hb in central pallor	Thalassemias (major, minor and intermedia), HbSC disease, liver disease, IDA, hyposplenism
Basophilic stippling (composed of RNA/ribosome)	Multiple granules in cytoplasm	Thalassemia, MDS, heavy metal poisoning, sideroblastic anemia, megaloblastic anemia
Howell-Jolly bodies (DNA)	Single dark blue like pyknotic nuclei	Hemolytic anemia, megaloblastic anemia, hyposplenic states
Cabot rings (mitotic spindle)	Ring or figure of 8	Megaloblastic anemia, hemolytic anemia
HbH inclusions	Golf ball appearance	Thalassemia, erythroleukemia
Heinz bodies (denatured hemoglobin)	Dot like structure seen on supravital stains	G6PD deficiency anemia
Pappenheimer bodies (iron)	Large blue like Howell-Jolly bodies but more than one	Post-splenectomy
Sideroblasts (iron)	Multiple granule of iron (seen after Prussian blue stain)	Sideroblastic anemia, MDS

Abbreviations: DNA, deoxyribonucleic acid; RNA, ribonucleic acid; HbSC, hemoglobin sickle cell; IDA, iron deficiency anemia; MDA, myelodysplastic syndrome; G6PD, glucose-6-phosphate dehydrogenase

6. Correct method of blood collection:

1. Fill forms
2. Identify the patient
3. See file
4. Bedside collection
5. Label the tubes

These options were jumbled in the examination as options. Correct order is:

1. Assemble equipment (needle, syringe and vacutainer tube)
2. Perform handwash
3. Identify and prepare the patient
4. Select the site
5. Apply torniquet 4–5 finger width above the selected venipuncture site
6. Ask the patient to form a fist so that veins are more prominent
7. Put on well fitting sterile gloves
8. Disinfect the site using 70% isoprophyl alcohol for 30 seconds
9. Enter the vein at 30 degree angle
10. Once sufficient blood has been collected, release the torniquet before withdrawing the needle
11. Discard the used needle and syringe
12. Check the label and amount for accuracy
13. Remove gloves and place them in the general waste.

7. All are reduced in iron deficiency anemia *except*:

A. Ferritin B. Total iron-binding capacity
C. Iron D. Transferrin

ANS. **B**

Total iron-binding capacity (TIBC) is increased in iron deficiency anemia (IDA), decreased in anemia of chronic diseases.

Differential diagnosis of microcytic anemia				
	Iron deficiency anemia	*Anemia of chronic disease*	*Thalassemia*	*Sideroblastic anemia*
MCV	Reduced	Low normal or normal	Low	Low inherited but normal in acquired
Serum iron	Reduced	Reduced	Normal	Raised
Serum TIBC	Raised	Reduced	Normal	Normal
Serum ferritin	Reduced	Normal or raised	Normal	Raised
Iron in BM	Absent	Present	Present	Present

Abbreviations: MCV, mean corpuscular volume; TIBC, total iron-binding capacity; BM, bone marrow

Stages of iron deficiency anemia

1. Stage of negative iron balance
   - Serum iron is normal
   - Serum TIBC increases

- Seum ferritin decreases
- Bone marrow iron decreases
- Percentage transferrin saturation is normal

2. Stage of iron deficient erythropoiesis
   - Serum iron decreases
   - Percentage transferrin saturation decreases
3. Stage of microcytic hypochromic anemia
   - Peripheral smear shows microcytic hypochromic anemia
   - Serum iron decreases
   - Percentage transferrin saturation decreases.

8. In breast cancer, fluorescence in situ hybridization (FISH) for gene amplification will be done based on which of the following immunohistochemistry (IHC) staining for HER2/neu?

A. 1 B. 2
C. 3 D. Any of the above

ANS. **B**

HER2/neu (ERB2) checks on membrane positivity and we look for percent of cells positive and intensity of positivity. Based on this, we classify HER2/neu results as:

- 0 or 1: negative
- 2: equivocal
- 3: positive

For an equivocal HER2/neu, we have to look for HER2/neu amplification by FISH.

Membrane positivity by HER2/neu

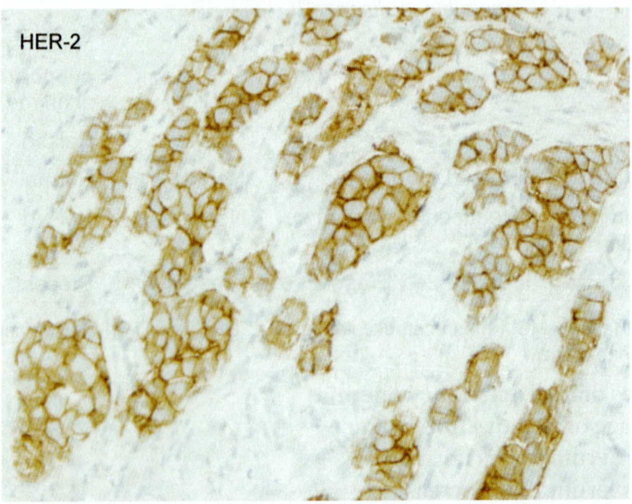

Estrogen receptor (ER)/progesterone receptor (PR) undergoes nuclear staining

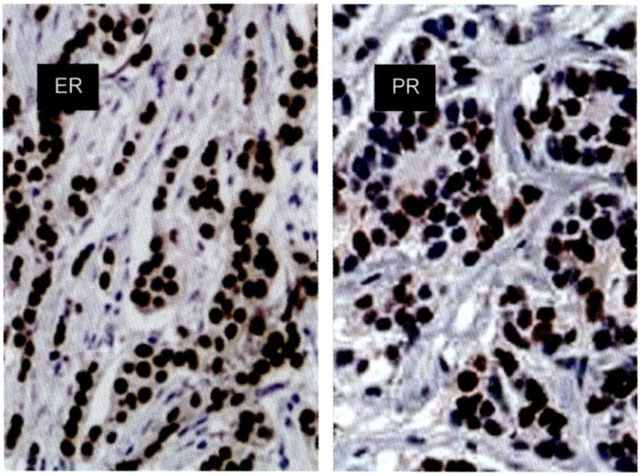

9. A depressed patient came with sudden onset of dyspnea. Chest X-ray (CXR) shows bilateral diffuse infiltrates with predominant involvement of right middle and lower lobes. He could not be saved despite treatment and on autopsy, the lungs appeared normal grossly. Histopathological examination (HPE) showed the following. What is the cause of death?

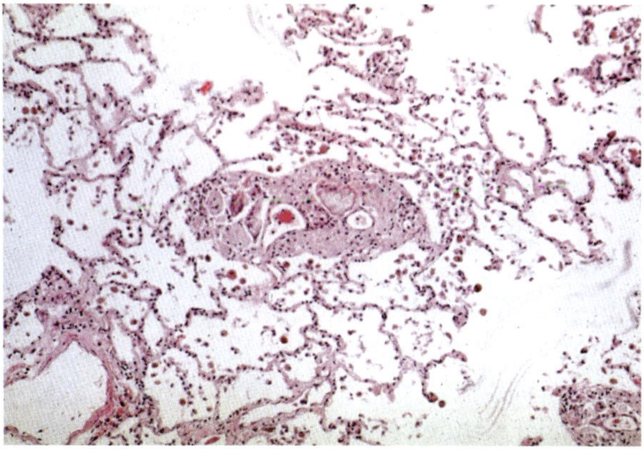

A. Necrotizing tuberculous (TB) granuloma
B. Vegetative matter (aspiration pneumonia)
C. Sarcoid granuloma
D. Severe fungal pneumonia

ANS. **B**

The given histopathological slide shows a granuloma with a refractile material indicative of foreign body.

The hints from the question are:

- A depressed lady
- Involvement of right middle and lower lobes (more prone for aspiration)
- Normal gross appearance of lungs.

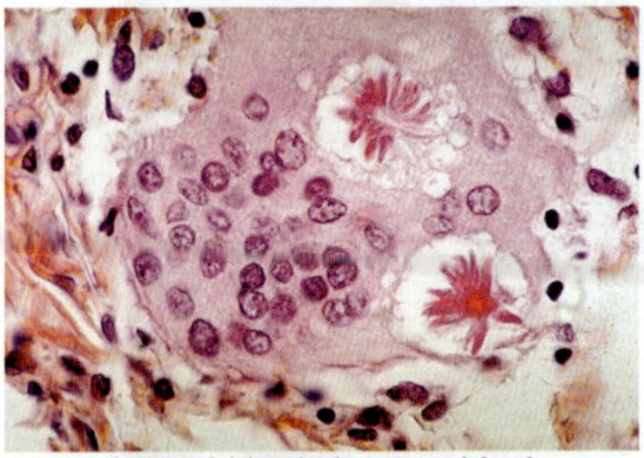

Asteroid body in sarcoidosis

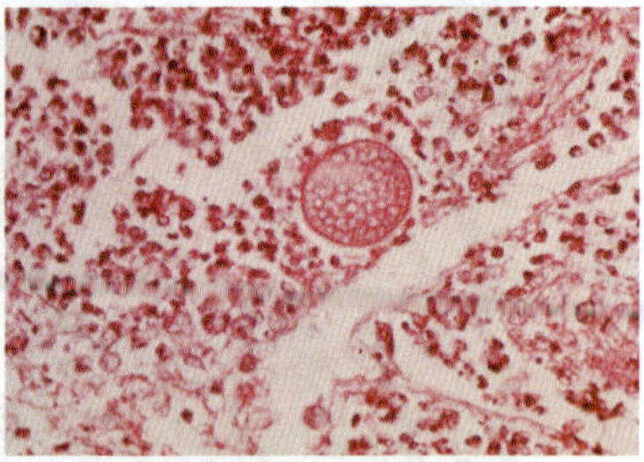

Coccidioidomycosis lung

Tuberculous granuloma

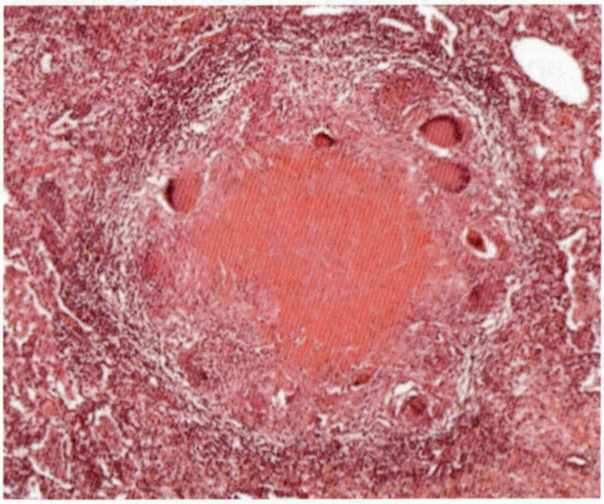

10. Origin of chronic lymphocytic leukemia (CLL)/small lymphocytic lymphoma (SLL)?

A. Centrocytes

B. Extranodal mature peripheral B cell

C. Naïve B cells in interfollicular zones

D. Bone marrow progenitors

ANS. **C**

B-cell chronic lymphocytic leukemia (**B-CLL**), also known as **chronic lymphoid leukemia** (**CLL**), is the most common type of leukemia in adults. CLL affects B-cell lymphocytes, which originate in the bone marrow, develop in the lymph nodes, and normally fight infection by producing antibodies.

Pathological findings in CLL

1. Smudge cells

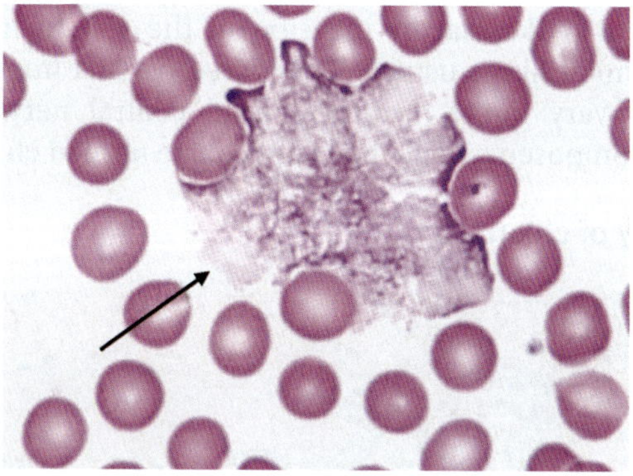

2. Pseudofollicles
3. Proliferation center
4. Convent girl appearance
5. CLL can produce warm hemolytic anemia
6. CLL transforming into diffuse large B-cell lymphoma (DLBCL) is called Ritcher's transformation.

Staging of CLL: Rai and Binnet staging

- Another hallmark is immunoglobulin variabll-region heavy-chain (IgVH) hypermutation and zeta-chain-associated protein (ZAP) 70 mutation
- Please know that ZAP 70 mutation has a poor prognosis on CLL.

11. A child with bilateral proptosis which investigation will help you in arriving at a diagnosis of chloroma?

A. Peripheral smear
B. Platelets
C. Hemoglobin concentration
D. Leukocyte count

ANS. **A**

A **chloroma** is an extramedullary manifestation of acute myeloid leukemia; in other words, it is a solid collection of leukemic cells occurring outside of the bone marrow.

Best way of diagnosing chloroma is PBS and biopsy of lesions

Currently, any extramedullary manifestation of acute myeloid leukemia can be termed a granulocytic sarcoma or chloroma. Specific terms which overlap with granulocytic sarcoma include:

- **Leukemia cutis,** describing infiltration of the dermis (skin) by leukemic cells, which is also referred to as cutaneous granulocytic sarcoma.
- **Meningeal leukemia,** or invasion of the subarachnoid space by leukemic cells, is usually considered distinct from chloroma, although very rarely occurring solid central nervous system tumors composed of leukemic cells can be termed chloromas.

Histology of chloroma

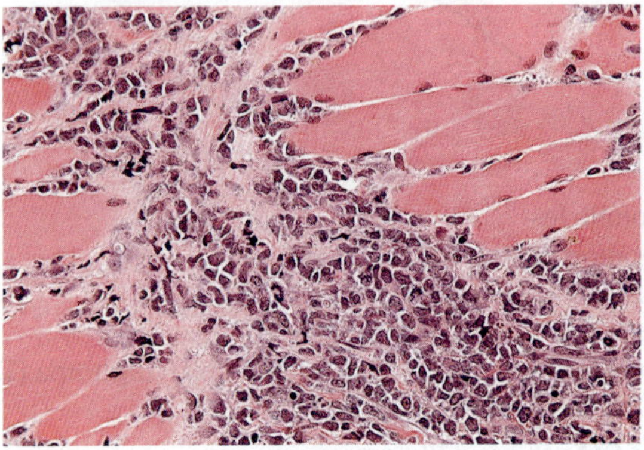

12. From a hilly area, male patient with fever and splenomegaly total leukocyte count (TLC) was 21,000, differential count showed metamyelocytes and myelocytes (around 40%). Hb was 16, lymphocytes were normal, platelets were normal, next investigation will be:

A. Erythropoietin estimation
B. Philadelphia chromosome
C. JAK2 mutations
D. Bone marrow biopsy with reticulin stain

ANS. **A**

Approach to polycythemia

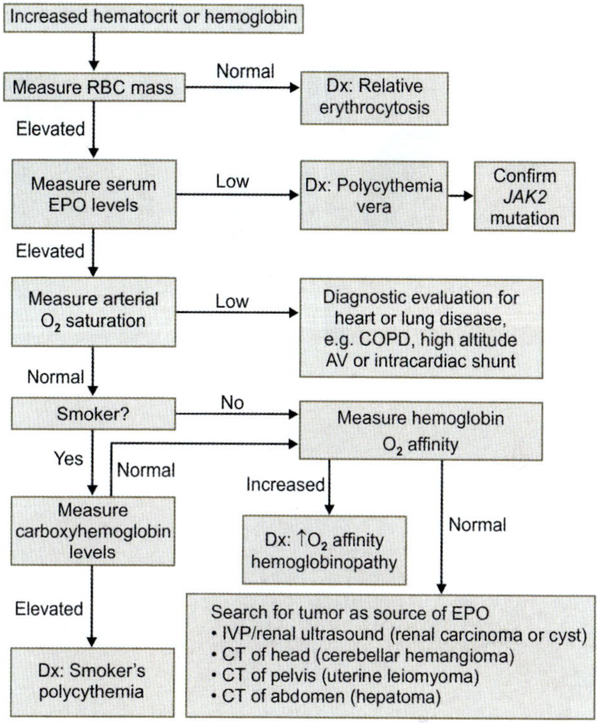

Abbreviations: RBC, red blood cell; EPO, erythropoietin; COPD, chronic obstructive pulmonary disease; IVP, intravenous pyelogram; CT, computed tomography

Criteria for Polycythemia

Major criteria:

- Hb >16.5 g/dL in males or Hb >16 g/dL in females or red cell mass >25% of previous value
- JAK2 V617 F mutation (valine changed to phenylalanine)
- Panmyelosis

Minor criteria:

EPO levels normal.

13. Endoscopic picture of a lesion in esophagus is shown below. What is the expected histopathology finding?

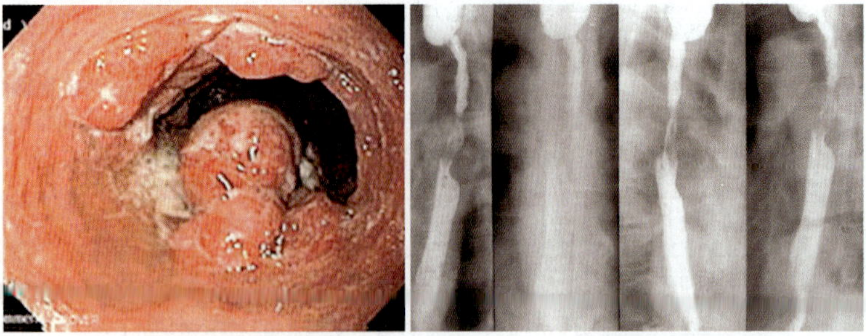

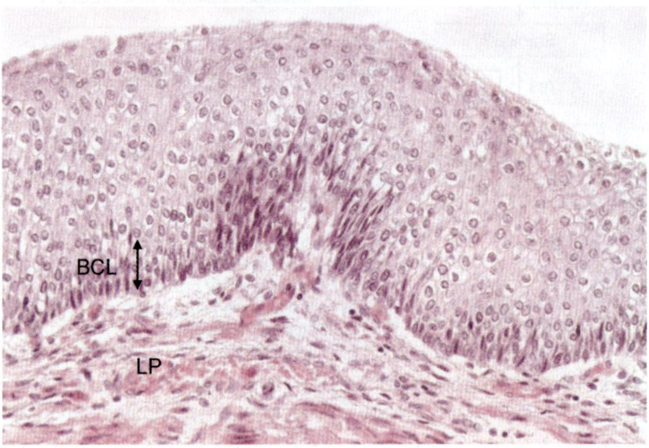

A.

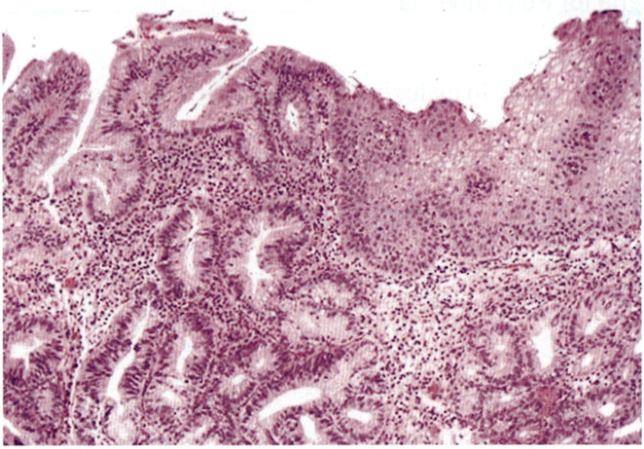

B.

C. 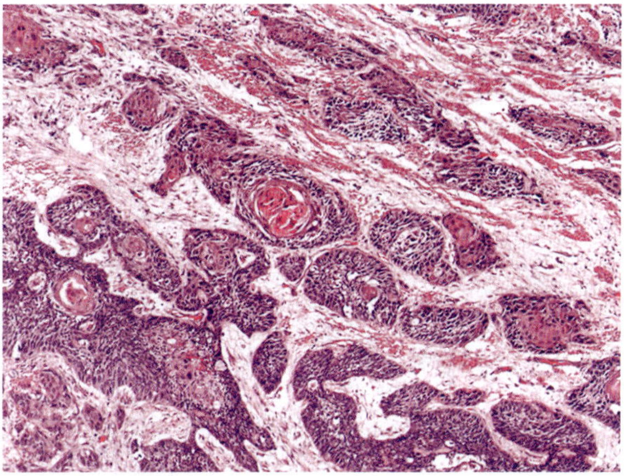

D. 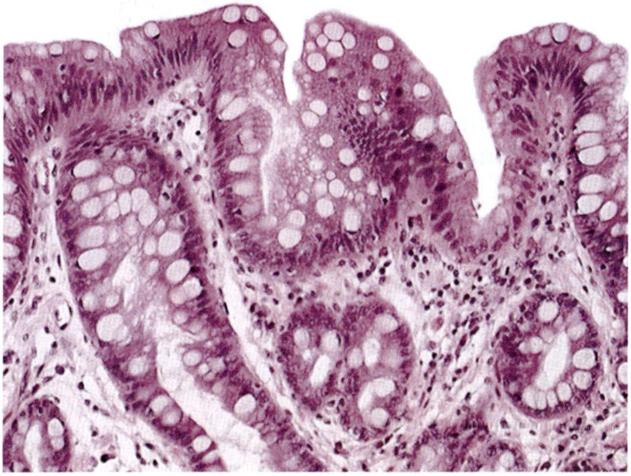

ANS. **C**

The endoscopy shows an exophytic lesion. Barium swallow shows a lesion at the middle 1/3rd of the esophagus.

Hence the diagnosis is squamous cell carcinoma esophagus.

Now let's go to the options.

- Option A shows a normal esophagus with stratified squamous epithelium
- Option B shows glandular pattern suggestive of adenocarcinoma
- Option C shows classical keratin pearls suggestive of squamous cell carcinoma
- Option D shows squamous metaplasia suggestive of Barrett's esophagus.

14. A 30-year-old male patient presented with dyspnea ECHO showed mitral stenosis with left atrial hypertrophy. Excised mitral valve is as shown. What is the diagnosis?

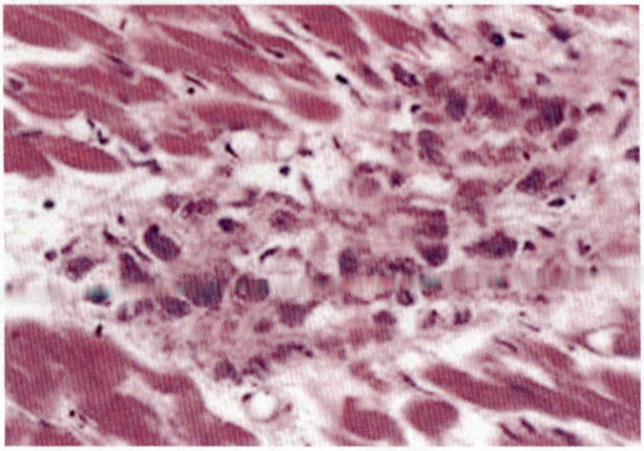

A. Tuberculosis
B. Sarcoidosis
C. Rheumatic heart diseases
D. Fungal granuloma

ANS. **C**

Vegetations in various conditions

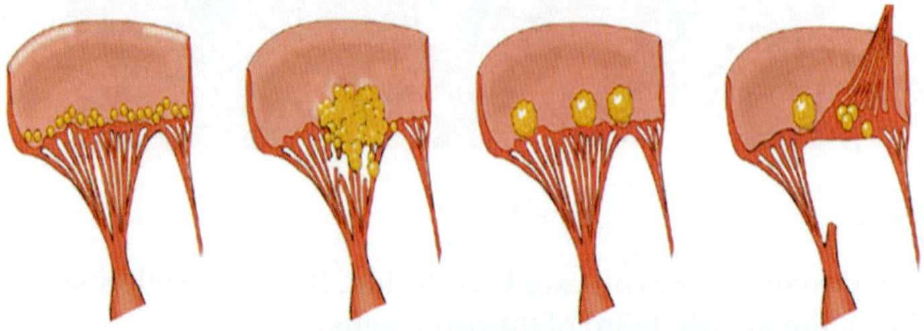

Another important question in cardiology is gross and microscopic changes in myocardial infarction (May AIIMS 2016)

Morphologic changes of myocardial infarction		
Time after onset	*Gross examination*	*Light microscopy*
4–12	No obvious change	Coagulation necrosis; edema; hemorrhage

Contd...

Contd...

<24	Dark mottling	Coagulation necrosis (eosinophilia) Pyknosis of nuclei and vacuolar degeneration "Wavy fibers"
1–3 days	Mottling with yellow-tan infarct center	Coagulation necrosis Loss of nuclei and striations Neutrophilic infiltration
3–7 days	Central yellow-tan softening with hyperemic border	Myofibers desolution Neutrophilic decrease Phagocytosis of dead cells by macrophages at infarct border
7–10 days	Depressed red-tan margins	Granulation tissue formation
10–14 days	Noticible infarct borders	Well-established granulation tissue with collagen deposition
2–8 weeks	Inward progression of scar	Increased collagen deposition with decreased cellularity
>2 months	Scarring complete	Dense collagenous scar

Microscopic features of myocardial infarction

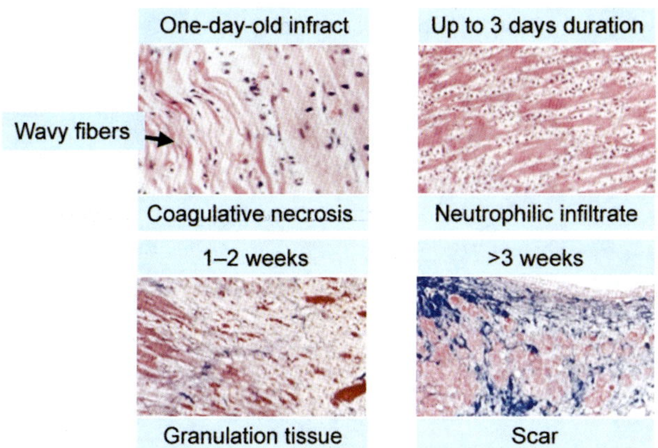

15. Best fixative for Pap smear:

A. 95% ethanol + 5% ether B. 10% formaldehyde
C. 80% isopropyl alcohol D. 90% ether + alcohol

ANS. **A**

Fixatives:

- Pap smear: 95% ethanol + 5% ether
- Light microscopy: 10% formaldehyde
- Electric microscopy: 2% glutaraldehyde
- For liquid-based cytology: Methanol
- For bone marrow biopsy: Zenker's fluid
- For bone marrow aspirate: Helly's fluid
- Cell block: Bouin's fluid
- Karyotyping fixatives: Carnoy's fixative (3:1 methanol to glacial acetic acid)
- Gastrointestinal biopsies: Bouin's fluid.

16. Serum lactate dehydrogenase (LDH) increased with normal alpha fetoprotein (AFP) is seen with:

A. Dysgerminoma B. Yolk sac tumor
C. Brenner's D. Mucinous cystodenocarcinoma

ANS. **A**

Histology slides of gynecological malignancies

Granulosa cell tumor (coffee bean nuclei)

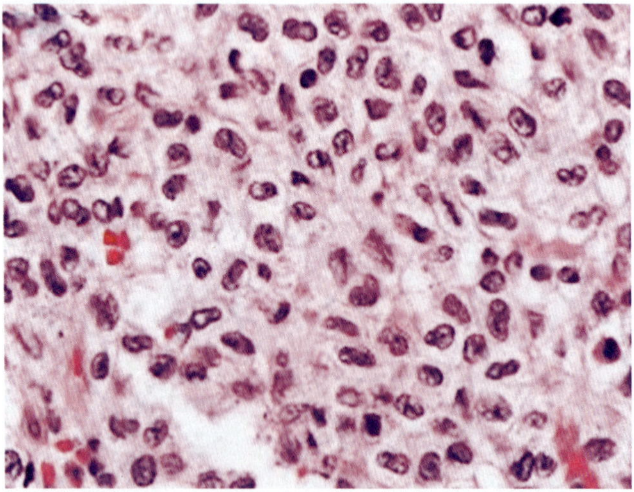

Yolk sac tumor

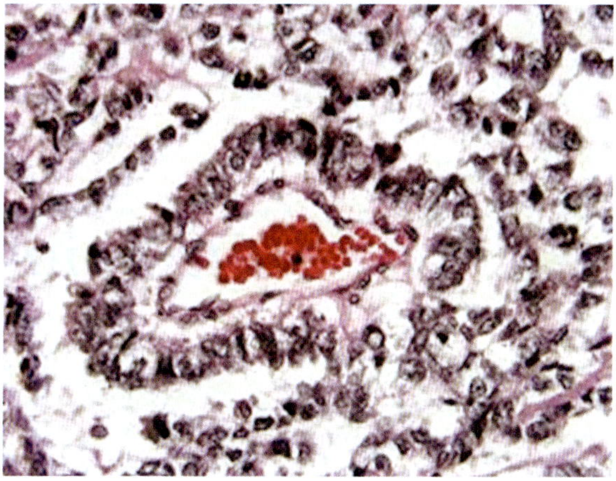

Krukenberg tumor (spindle cells)

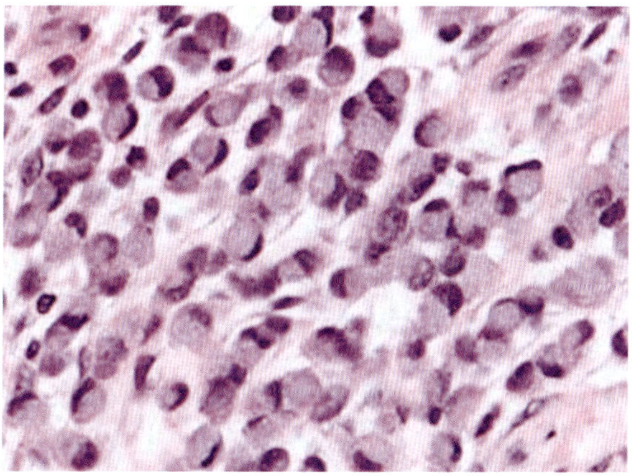

5

CHAPTER

Microbiology

1. Relapse is seen in which malaria?

1. *P. vivax* 2. *P. falciparum*
3. *P. malariae* 4. *P. ovale*
A. 1 and 2 B. 2 and 3
C. 3 and 4 D. 1 and 4

ANS. **D**

	P. falciparum	*P. vivax*	*P. ovale*	*P. malariae*
Tissue schizogony	5–6 days	8 days	9 days	13 days
Erythrocytic phase	48 hours	48 hours (benign tertain)	49–50 hours (ovale tertian)	72 hours (quartan)
Red cells affected	All	Reticulocytes	Reticulocytes	Mature RBCs
Hypnozoites	No	Yes	Yes	No, but blood forms can persist up to 30 years
Incubation period in humans	12 days	13–17 days	13–17 days	28–30 days
Pigmentation	Maurer's	Schuffner's	James'	Ziemann's

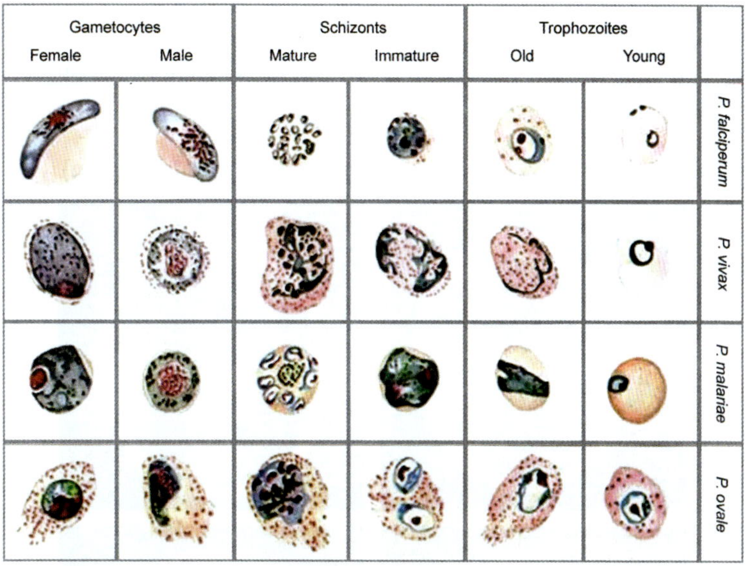

2. Not a dimorphic fungi?

A. *Histpolasma* B. *P. jiroveci*
C. *Sporothrix* D. Blastomycosis

ANS. **B**

Dimorphic fungi are fungi which can exist as mold/hyphal/ filamentous form or as yeast.

Examples of dimorphic fungi (HSBC) + P

1. *Histoplasma* 2. *Sporothrix*
3. Blastomycosis 4. Coccidiomycosis
5. *Penicillium*

3. Neonatal CMV is best diagnosed from:

A. CSF B. Urine
C. Blood D. Liver biopsy

ANS. **B**

- Best diagnosis of neonatal CMV is from saliva > urine.
- Since saliva is not given as options, the best answer is urine.

Congenital CMV infection

Presentation

1. Low birth weight
2. Microcephaly

3. Seizures
4. Periventricular calcification
5. Petechial rash similar to blueberry muffin (congenital rubella)
6. Hepatosplenomegaly.

MRI finding in CMV infection (periventricular calcification)

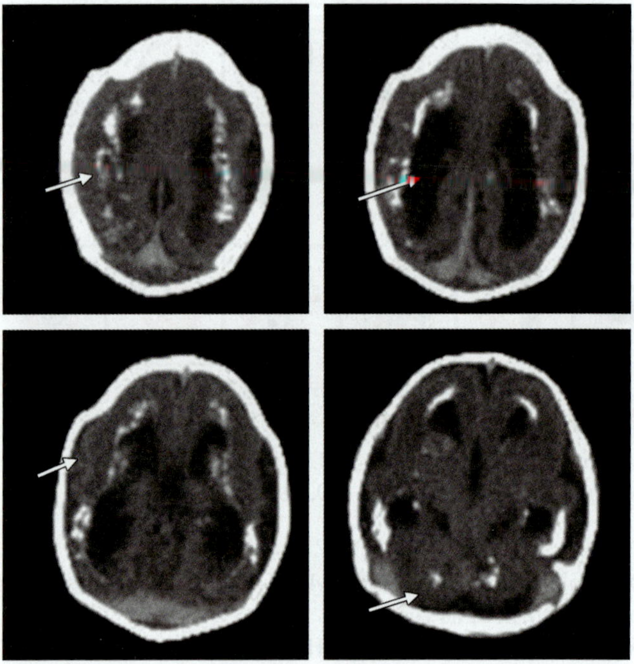

Inclusion body in CMV (Owl's eye appearance)

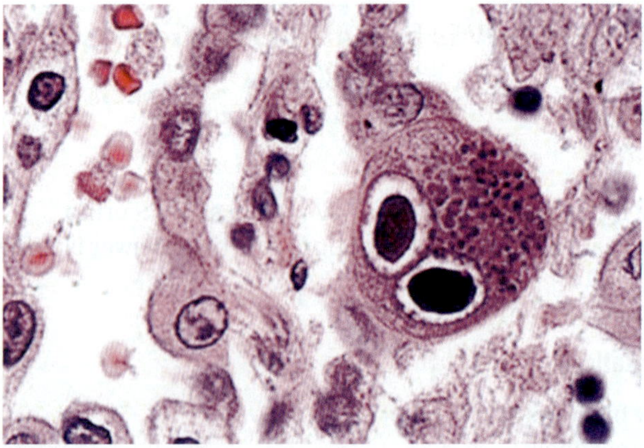

4. Blood spill disinfection by:

A. Isopropyl alcohol
B. Hypochlorite
C. Formalin
D. Glutaraldehyde

ANS. **B**

Spaulding's classification for sterilization

1. Critical, e.g. heart lung machine, scalpel (contact with blood)
2. Semicritical, e.g. endoscopes
3. Noncritical, e.g. stethoscope, BP cuff, plasters.

Method of sterilization

1. Critical: Autoclave/ethylene oxide
2. Semicritical: 2% glutaraldehyde for 20 minutes
3. For plastic tubes: Gamma rays

5. 1,3 beta-D glucan assay is used in the diagnosis of:

A. Tuberculosis
B. *Histoplasma*
C. Invasive candidiasis
D. *Cryptococcus*

ANS. **C**

β-glucans (beta-glucans) comprise a group of β-D-glucose polysaccharides naturally occurring in the cell walls of cereals, bacteria, and fungi, with significantly differing physicochemical properties dependent on source.

An assay to detect the presence of (1, 3)-β-D-glucan in blood is marketed as a means of identifying invasive candidiasis.

Caspofungin

This is the latest antifungal, belonging to the group, Echinocandins, which blocks beta 1,3 glucan synthase.

6. Lipoarabinomannan assay (LAM):

A. *M. tuberculosis*
B. *Cryptococcus*
C. *Listeria*
D. *Pneumococcus*

ANS. **A**

Newer targets used for diagnosing tuberculosis

1. **Lipoarabinomannan**, also called LAM, is a glycolipid, and a virulence factor associated with *Mycobacterium tuberculosis*, the bacteria responsible for tuberculosis. Its primary function is to inactivate macrophages and scavenge oxidative radicals.

The inactivation of macrophages allows for the dissemination of mycobacteria to other parts of the body. The destruction of oxidative radicals allows for the survival of the bacteria, as oxidative free radicals are an important mechanism by which our bodies try to rid ourselves of infection.

2. ESAT-6, the 6 kDa early secretory antigenic target produced by *Mycobacterium tuberculosis,* is a secretory protein and potent T cell antigen. It is used in tuberculosis diagnosis by the whole blood interferon γ test QuantiFERON-TB Gold.
3. CFP-10 is a 10 kDa secreted antigen from *Mycobacterium tuberculosis.* It forms a 1:1 heterodimeric complex with ESAT-6. Both genes are expressed from the RD1 region of the bacterial genome and play a key role in the virulence of the infection.

7. Diagnosis of *Cl. difficile* diagnosis:

A. Toxin gene detection by polymerase chain reaction (PCR)
B. Culture
C. Enzyme-linked immunosorbent assay (ELISA)
D. Nagler's reaction

ANS. **A**

Clostridium difficile associated colitis (pseudomembranous enterocolitis)

- Most common antibiotic associated with pseudomembranous enterocolitis: Third generation cephalosporin
- Most prone antibiotic: Clindamycin

Endoscopic image of pseudomembrane

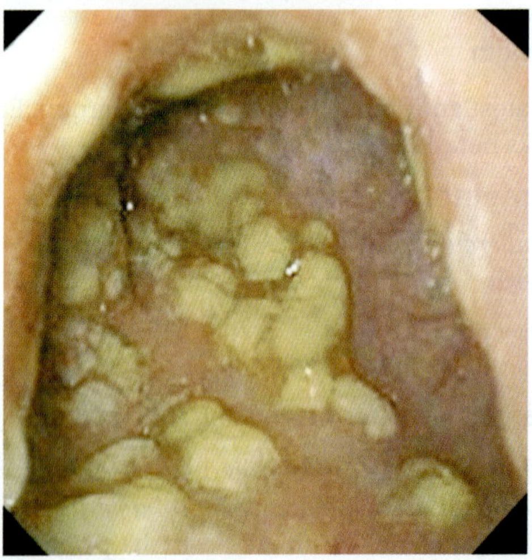

CT image of pseudomembranous enterocolitis

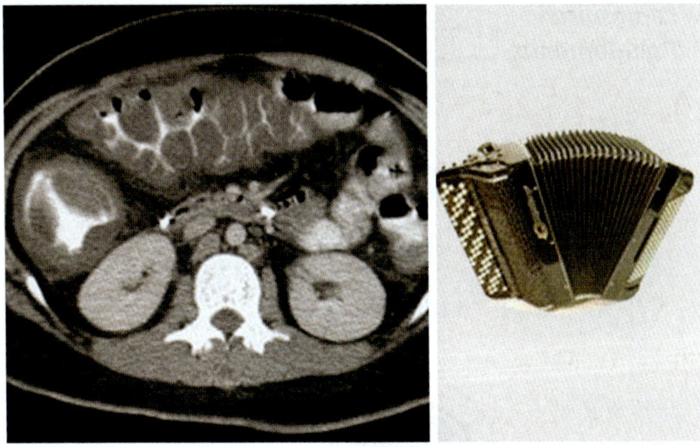

8. Recently confirmed viral case in India:

A. Yellow fever B. Crimean-Congo fever
C. Ebola virus D. Zika virus

ANS. **B**

Crimean-Congo hemorrhagic fever (CCHF) is a viral disease.

Symptoms may include fever, muscle pains, headache, vomiting, diarrhea, and bleeding into the skin. Onset of symptoms is less than two weeks following exposure.

Complications may include liver failure. In those who survive, recovery generally occurs around two weeks after onset.

The CCHF virus is typically spread by *tick bites* or contact with livestock carrying the disease.

Diagnosis is by detecting antibodies, the virus's RNA, or the virus itself.

Prevention involves avoiding tick bites. A vaccine is not commercially available. Treatment is typically with supportive care.

The medication ribavirin may also help.

CCHF in India

In India the first confirmed case of CCHF was reported during a nosocomial (Infections caught in hospitals) outbreak in Ahmadabad, Gujarat, in January 2011. Subsquently outbreaks were reported from different districts of Gujarat every year. During 2012-2015, several outbreaks and cases of CCHF transmitted by ticks via livestock and several nosocomial infections were reported in the states of Gujarat and Rajasthan.

9. The following structure is seen in:

A. *Leptospira* B. *Listeria*
C. *Pseudomonas* D. *H. pylori*

ANS. **A**

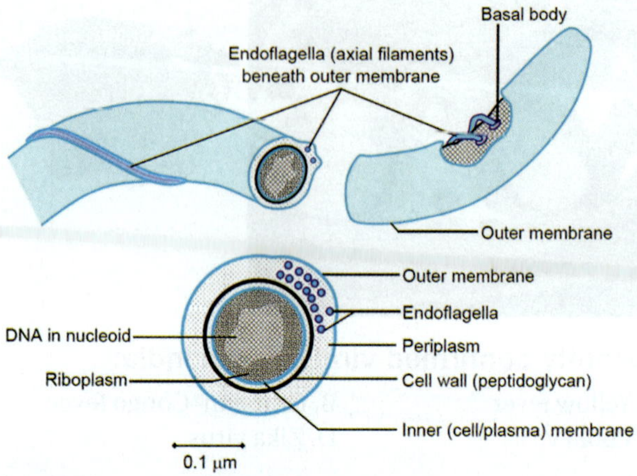

Different types of flagella:

1. Monotrichous flagella: *Vibrio, Pseudomonas*
2. Lophotrichous: *H. pylori*
3. Amphitrichous: *Spirella, C. jejuni*
4. Peritrichous: *E. coli, Proteus, Salmonella*

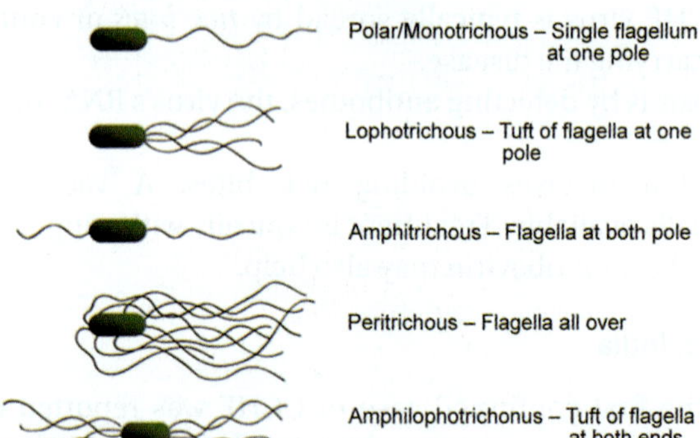

10. The following picture depicts which virus:

A. Hepatitis B B. Human immunodeficiency virus
C. Cytomegalovirus D. Herpes simplex

ANS. **A**

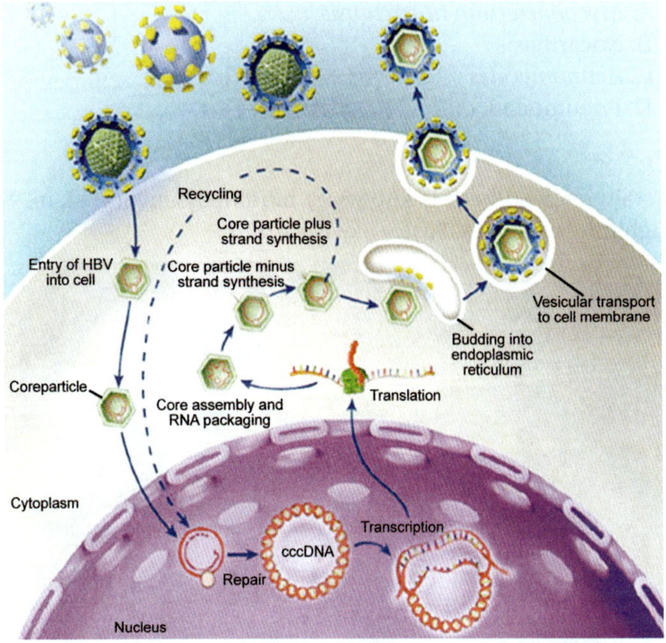

11. Identify the organism

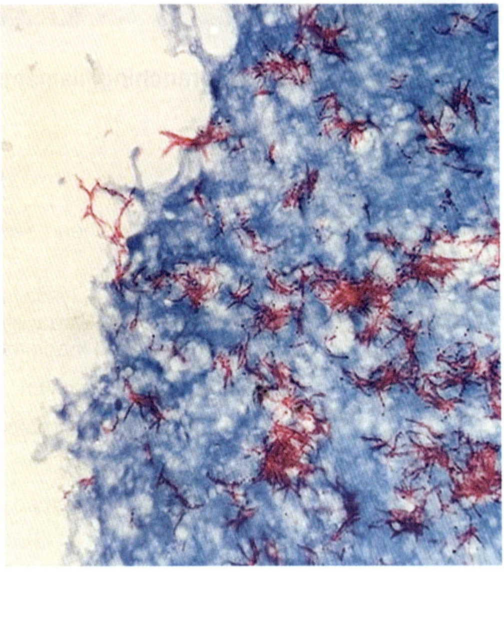

A. *Mycobacterium tuberculosis*
B. Nocardiasis
C. *Actinomycetes*
D. Pneumocooci

ANS. **A**

The stain showed here is known as modified Kinyoun stain. Even though this resembles closely like *Nocardia*.

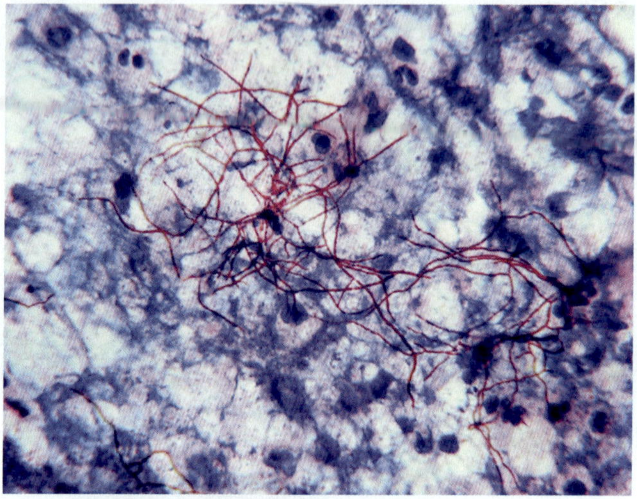

Nocardia is filamentous acid-fast branching filaments

Important culture medium

Organism	*Medium*
Bacillus cereus	Mannitol, yolk, phenol red agar (MYPA)
Bacillus anthracis	PLET (polymyxin, lysozyme, ethylenediaminetetraacetic acid, thallium acetate) medium
Bordetella	Bordet Gengou medium
Brucella	Castaneda method of blood culture
Campylobacter jejuni	Skirrow's
Chlamydiae	Tissue culture (irradiated McCoy cells, HeLa cells
Clostridia (anaerobic organisms)	Robertson's cooked meat broth, Thioglycollate, Smith Noguchi

Contd...

Contd...

Corynebacterium diphtheriae	Potassium tellurite blood agar
Legionella	Buffered charcoal yeast extract (BCYE)
Listeria	PALCAM (polymyxin acriflavin lithium chloride ceftazimide aesculin mannitol) agar
Leptospira	EMJH medium; Fletcher medium; Korthof medium
Mycobacterium tuberculosis	Lowenstein Jensen (LJ) medium Middle Brook's medium, Dorset Egg medium
Mycoplasma	PPLO (pleuropneumonia-like organism) medium
Neisseria gonorrhoeae	Thayer Martin medium and Chacko Nair medium
Pseudomonas	Cetrimide agar
Rickettsiae	Yolk sac of developing chick embryo
Salmonella	Wilson Blair medium
Shigella	Deoxycholate citrate agar
Spirochetes	Noguchi's medium
Streptococcus	Polymyxin, neomycin, fusidic acid
Staphylococcus	Ludlam's medium, Baird Parker agar, mannitol salt agar
Trypanosomes	Novy-Macneal-Nicolle medium

12. Fecal stain shown below is typical of:

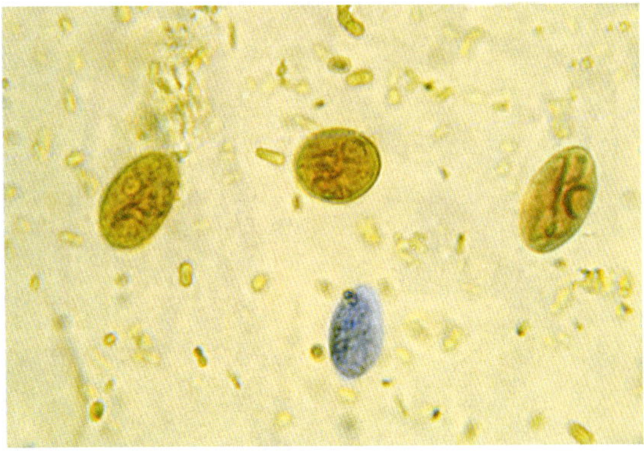

A. *Balantidum coli* B. *G.intestinalis*
C. *Ancyclostoma duodenale* D. *Enterobius vermicularis*

ANS. **B**

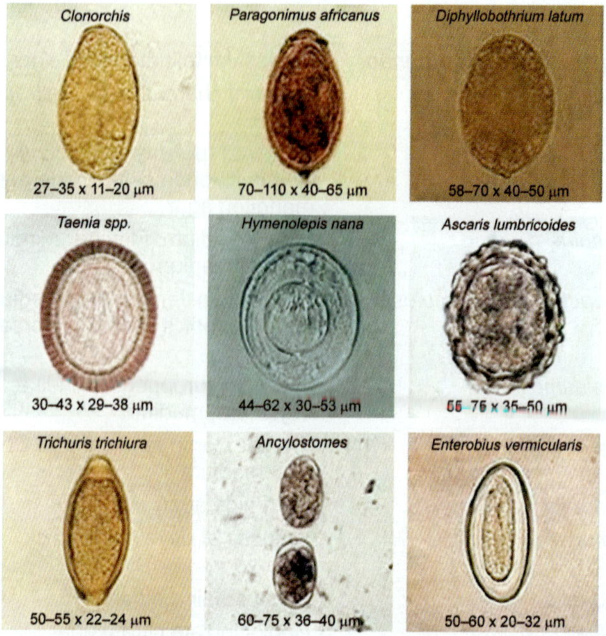

13. The organism shown below is:

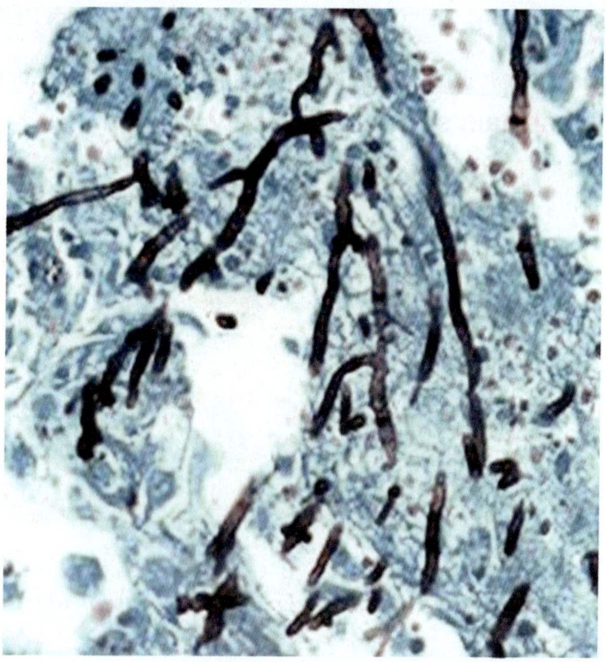

A. *Aspergillus* B. *Candida*
C. *Histoplasma* D. *Paracoccidiomycosis*

ANS. **A (Aspergillus has septations and it has acute branching)**

- ***Histoplasma* (feathery finger like projections)**

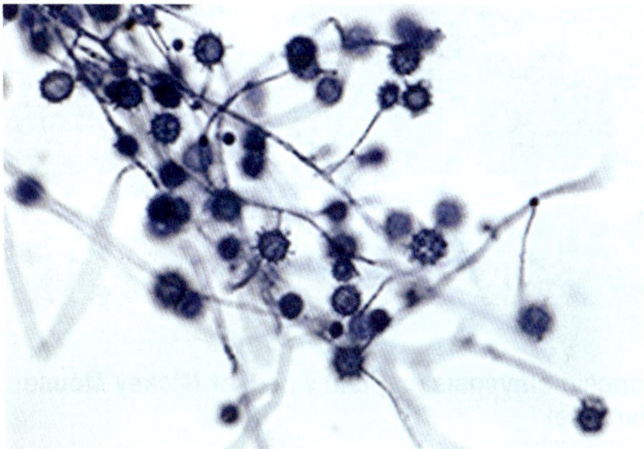

- **Blastomycosis (figure of 8 appearance)**

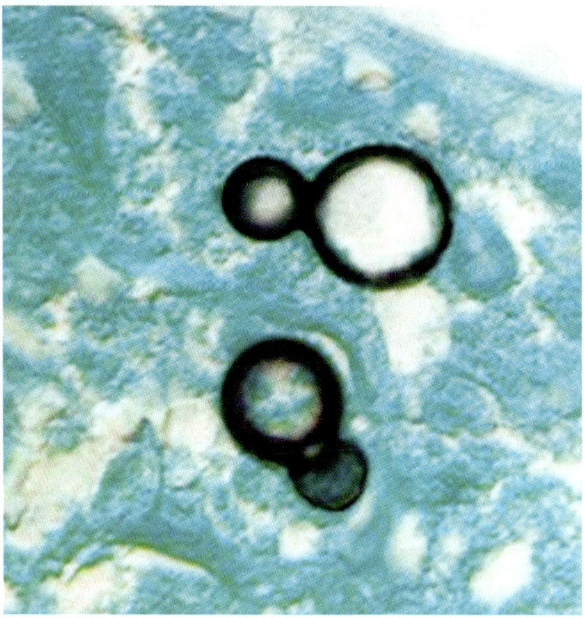

■ **Coccidiomycosis (spherules with spores)**

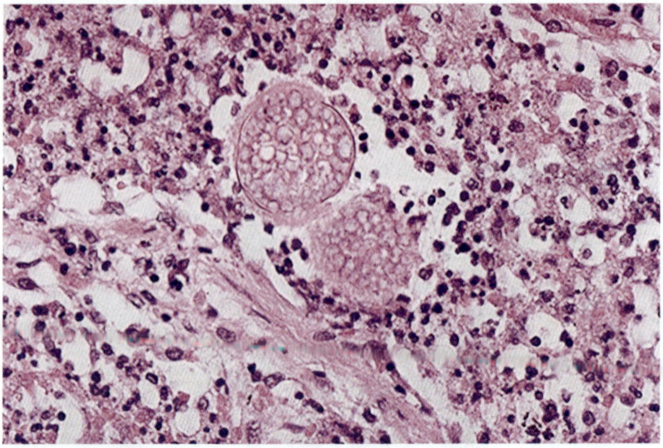

■ **Paracoccidiomycosis (captain wheel or Mickey Mouse appearance)**

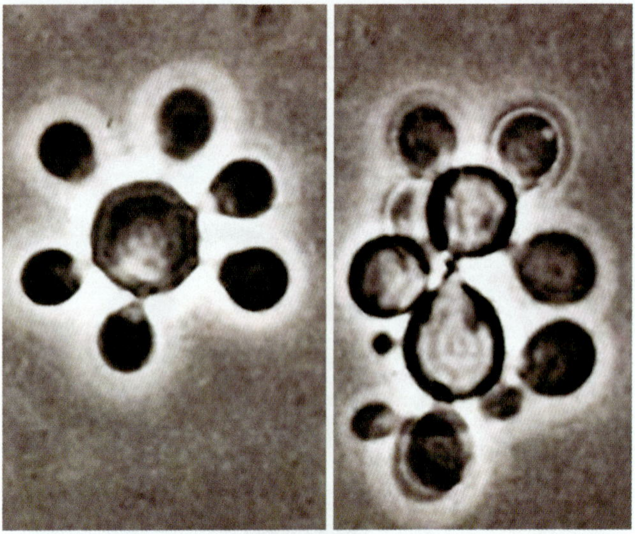

■ *Cryptococcus* (negative staining, polysaccharide capsule)

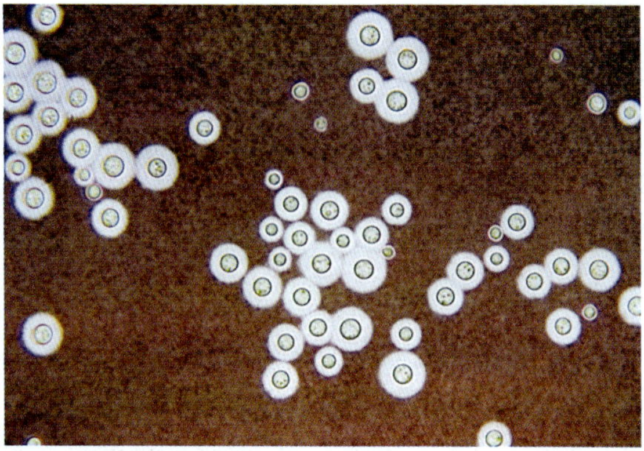

■ *Sporothrix schenki* (Flower shaped conidia and cigar bundles)

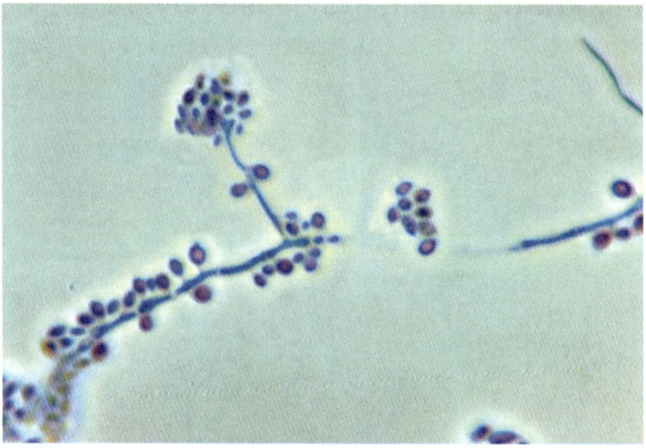

■ *Candida albicans* (germ tube formation)

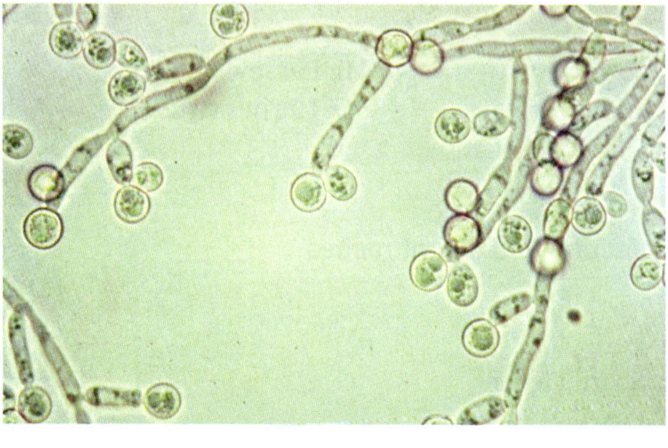

- ***Pneumocystis carinii* (Gomori methanamine stain, cup-shaped cyst)**

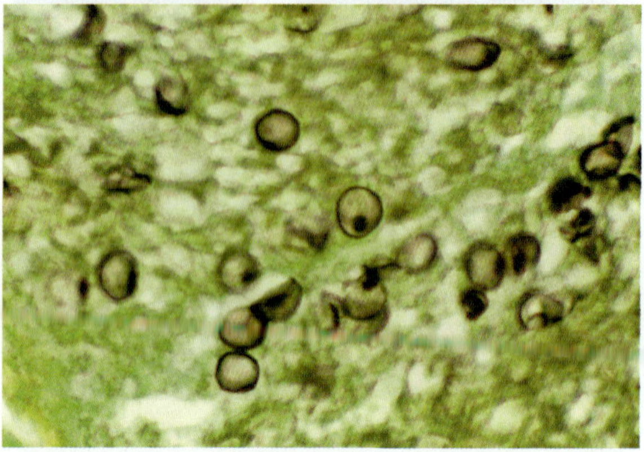

14. The following disease is caused by:

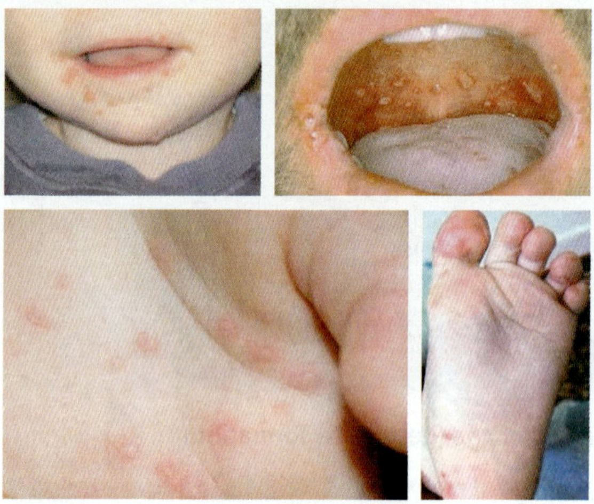

A. Coxsackie
B. Parvovirus B_{19}
C. Paramyxovirus
D. Herpes virus

ANS. **A**

- **Viral infection and day of rashes**

Rash on:

- Day 1: Varicella
- Day 2: Scarlet fever
- Day 3: Pox

- Day 4: Measles
- Day 5: Typhus
- Day 6: Dengue
- Day 7: Typhoid.

Shapes of viruses

1. Pox: Brick shaped
2. Adenovirus: Space vehicle
3. Rabies: Bullet shaped

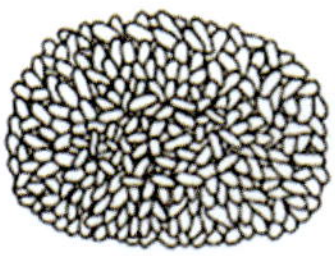

Poxviridae

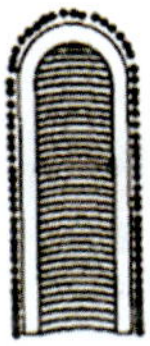

Rhabdviridae

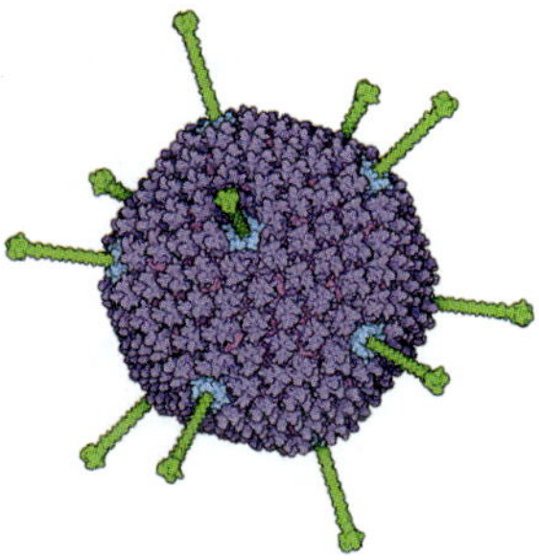

Measles

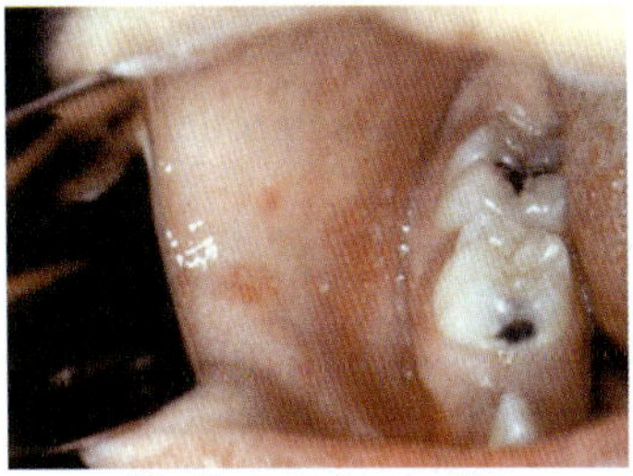

Koplik spots in measles

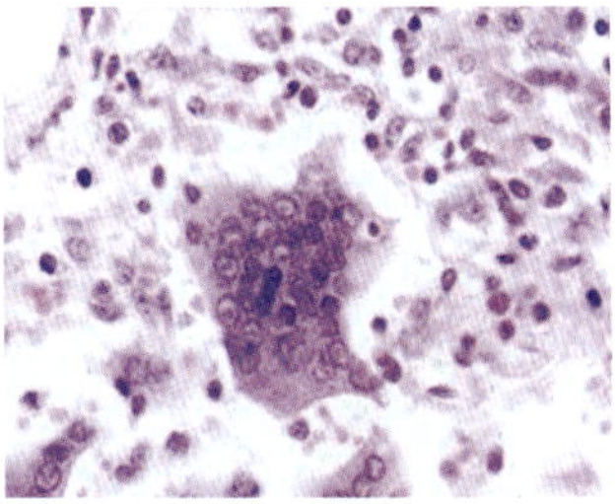

Warthin finkeldy giant cells

Slapped cheek syndrome (parvovirus B_{19})

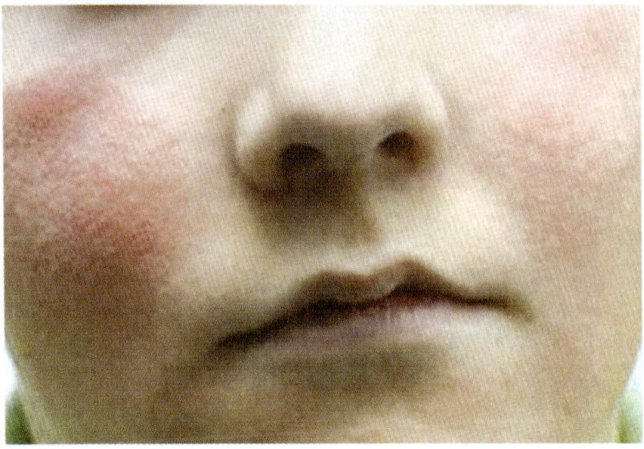

15. A farmer residing at Himachal Pradesh, developed a verrucous lesion following a thorn prick injury. Histopathological examination of the lesion showed the following. What is the diagnosis?

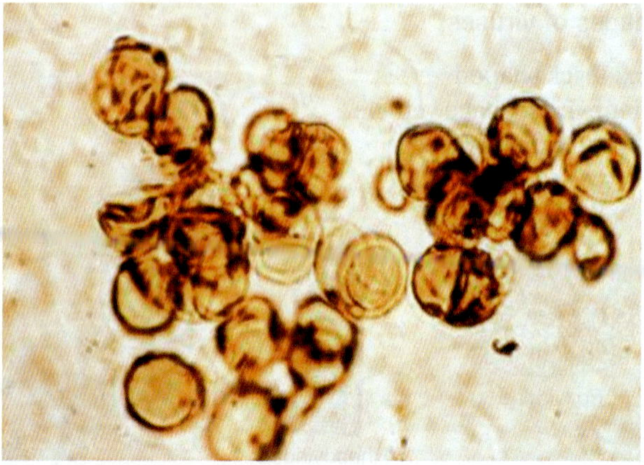

A. Sporotrichosis
B. Chromoblastomycosis
C. Brucellosis
D. Actinomycosis

ANS: **B**

- **Chromoblastomycosis with Medlar bodies/sclerotic/copper penny/muriform bodies**

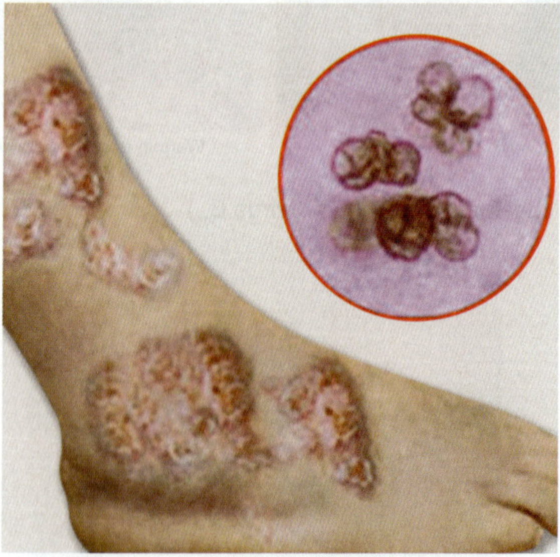

6
CHAPTER

Forensic Medicine and Toxicology

1. A person was bought to the casualty brought dead and autopsy was performed to find the cause of death. On external examination, only finding found was a mark on the chin as in 1st picture. And on internal examination of neck, there was a finding on anterior aspect of neck as shown below. What is the possible cause of death?

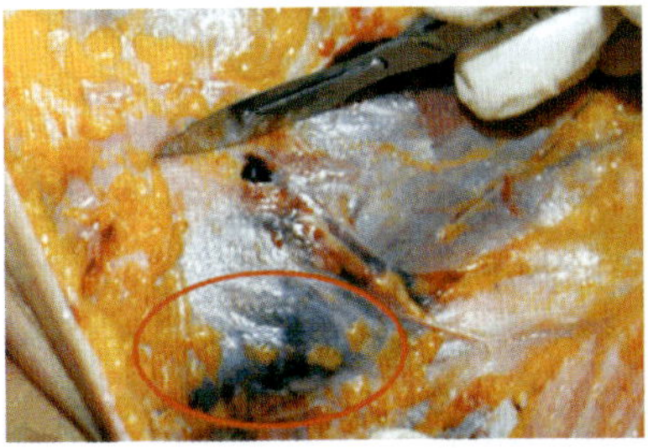

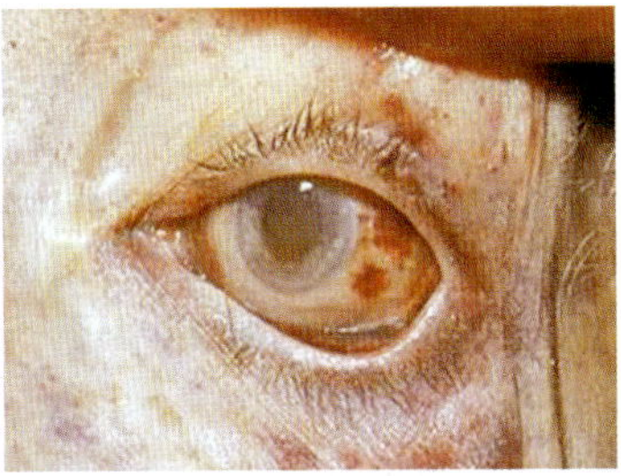

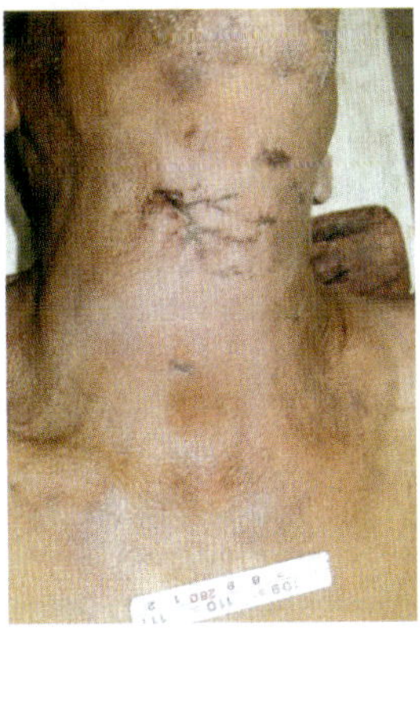

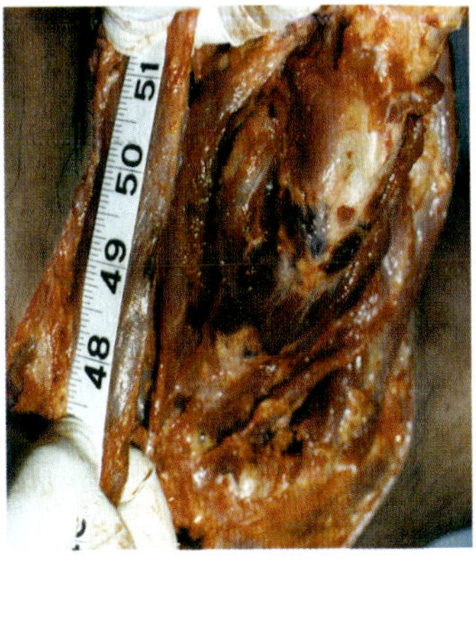

A. Throttling
B. Strangulation
C. Mugging
D. Hanging

ANS. **A**

Trait	*Hanging*	*Ligature strangulation*
Ligature strand	It is oblique; does not completely encircle the neck	It is transverse, completely encircling the neck
Subcutaneous tissues	White, hard and glistening under the mark	Ecchymosed under the mark
Face	Usually pale and petechiae are not common	Congested, bluish, and marked with petechiae
Bleeding	From the nose, mouth and ears are not common	From the nose, mouth and ears are common
Seminal fluid	At glans is more common	At glans is less common
Emphysematous bullae	Not present in the surface of lungs	Very common in surface of lungs
Carotid arteries	Damage may be seen	Damage is rare
Thyroid cartilage	Fracture is less common	Fracture is more common
Hyoid bone	Fracture is more common	Fracture is less common

2. Match the following:

1. Geneva — a. Torture
2. Tokyo — b. Abortion
3. Oslo — c. Human experimentation
4. Helsinki — d. Ethics

A. 1 = a, 2 = b, 3 = c, 4 = d
B. 1 = b, 2 = c, 3 = d, 4 = a
C. 1 = d, 2 = a, 3 = b, 4 = c
D. 1 = c, 2 = d, 3 = a, 4 = b

ANS. **C**

Declaration of Geneva	Modernized version of Hippocratic oath
Declaration of Helsinki	Human experimentation and clinical trials
Declaration of Sydney	Definition of death and recovery of organs
Declaration of Oslo	Therapeutic (legalized) abortion

Declaration of Munich	Discrimination in medicine
Declaration of Tokyo	Torture and medicine
Declaration of Lisbon	Right of patients
Declaration of Venice	Terminal illness
Declaration of Malta	Role of doctors in hunger strikes
Declaration of Istanbul	Organ trafficking and transplant tourism

3. Match the following:

1. Cocaine — a. Human hand
2. LSD — b. White lady
3. Abrus — c. Purple haze
4. Capsaicin — d. Gunchin

A. 1 = a, 2 = b, 3 = c, 4 = d B. 1 = b, 2 = c, 3 = d, 4 = a
C. 1 = d, 2 = a, 3 = b, 4 = c D. 1 = c, 2 = d, 3 = a, 4 = b

ANS. **B**

Cocaine: White lady

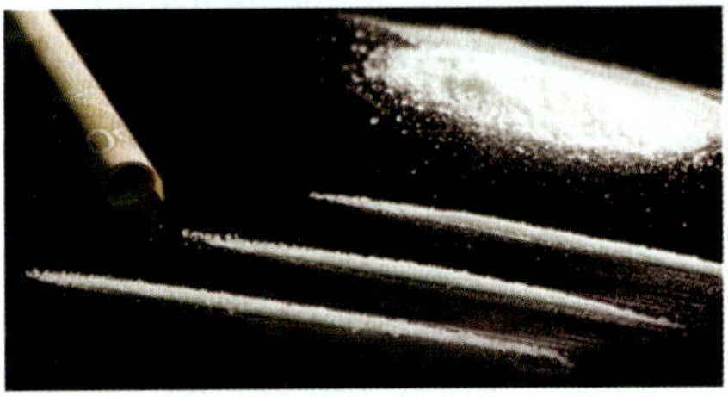

LSD: Purple haze

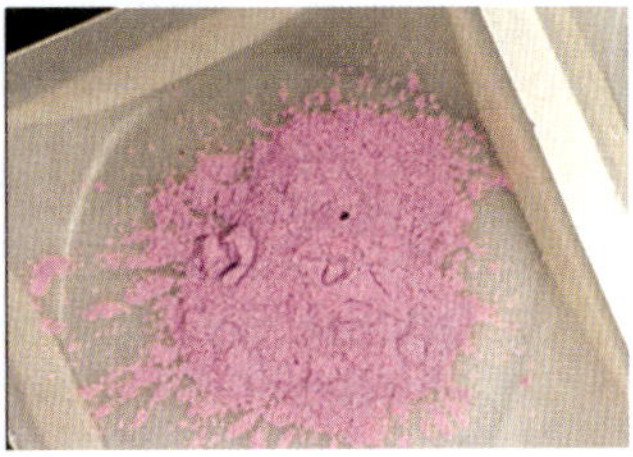

4. A 14-year-old victim of rape coming with 22 weeks pregnancy, what should not be done?

A. Male doctor can examine in the presence of female attendants
B. No need for vaginal swab
C. No need to confirm pregnancy
D. Can do termination of pregnancy with her consent by gynecologist

ANS. **D**

Pregnancy above 20 weeks cannot be terminated.

As per consent rules, child below 18 years cannot give consent to harm like MTP (87 IPC).

Important IPCs	
Laws related to consent	
Section 53 CrPc	In criminal cases as arrested person examined by the doctor without his consent and even using force
Section 54 CrPc	Arrested person can also request to be examined by a doctor to detect any evidence
Section 87 IPC	A person >18 years of age can give consent to suffer any harm if the act is not intended and not known to cause death or grievous hurt
Section 89 IPC	A child <12 years of age a person of unsound mind cannot give consent to suffer any harm
Section 90 IPC	Consent given by an insane person or given under fear of injury, death etc. or due to misconception of a fact is invalid
Section 92 IPC	Any harm caused to a person in good faith even without the person's consent is not an offence if the circumstances were such that it was impossible to obtain consent of the person or his lawful guardian at that material time for that thing to be done for the benefit of the person.

5. Correct order of Nysten's rule:

A. Orbicularis oculi, facial muscles, jaw, upper limb
B. Orbicularis oculi, facial muscles, upper limb, thorax
C. Muscles of eyelid, neck, upper limb, thorax
D. Muscles of eyelid, facial muscles, thorax, upper limb

ANS. **D**

Order of appearance of rigor mortis

1. Muscles of eyelids (3–5 hours)
2. Jaw, facial muscles (4–5 hours)
3. Neck, thorax (5–7 hours)
4. Upper limb (shoulder to hand): 7–9 hours
5. Abdomen, lower limb: 9–11 hours
6. Small muscles of fingers and toes: 11–12 hours.

Graph showing changes after death with time

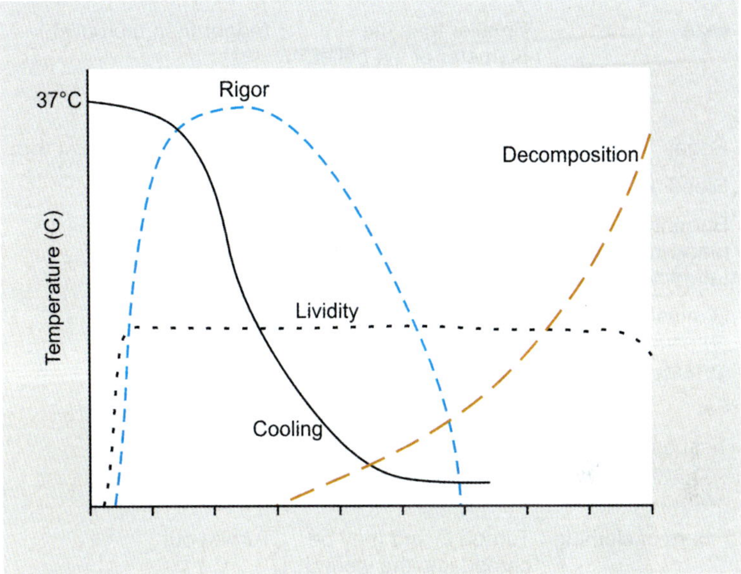

6. Atropine is not used in the poisoning of:

A. Parathion
B. Endrin
C. Tik 20
D. Baygon

ANS. **B**

Endrin is an organochlorine compound whereas all the others are organophosphorus compounds in which atropine is the specific antidote.

7. In the case of gun-shot injury to skull with entry wound surrounded by abrasion collar and tattooing and an exit wound along with metal fragments of bullet inside the bullet track, what will be preserved for calculating the range of firing?

A. Hair
B. Bullet pieces
C. Blood
D. Clothes

ANS. **A**

Hair should be analyzed for presence of any singering or smoke deposits.

Clothes can also be used, since skull is mentioned appropriate answer is hair.

Trait	*Entrance wound*	*Exit wound*
Size	Smaller than the diameter of the bullet. In close discharge, skin is torn	Bigger than the bullet
Edges	Inverted	Everted, puckered or torn
Bleeding	Less	More
Burning, blackening, tattooing	May be seen around the wound	Absent
Contusion, abrasion and grease collar	Present	Absent
Fat	No protrusion	May protrude
Tissues within and around the wound	May be cherry-red due to carbon monoxide of explosive gases	Absent
Fibers of clothing	Turned in and may be carried into the wound	Turned out
Lead ring or metal ring	May be seen around the wound by radiological examination	Absent
Spectrography	More metal is found around entrance wound, if bullet has only passed through soft tissues	The exit wound may contain more metal if a bone is struck nearer to it

8. Criminal responsiblity of insane is defined in:

A. McNaughton's rule　　B. Curren's rule
C. Durham rule　　D. American law institute test

ANS. **A**

9. Black foot is seen in which poisoning?

A. As　　B. Hg
C. Cu　　D. Ag

ANS. **A**

Arsenic poisoning black foot

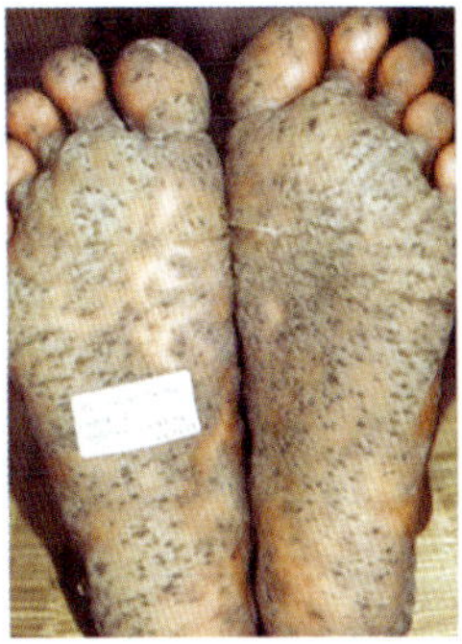

Aldrich-Mees' lines

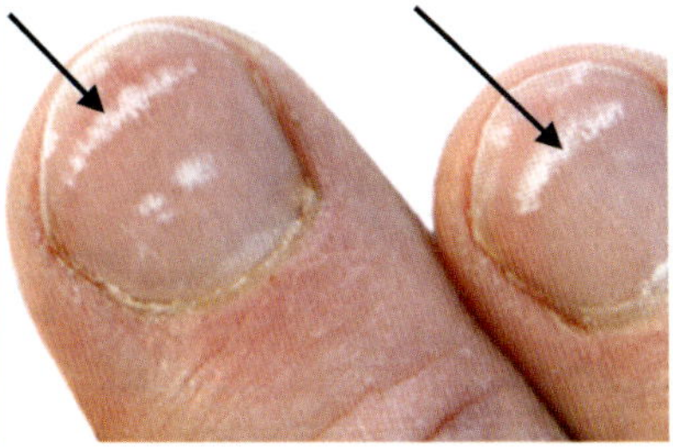

Rain drop pigmentation

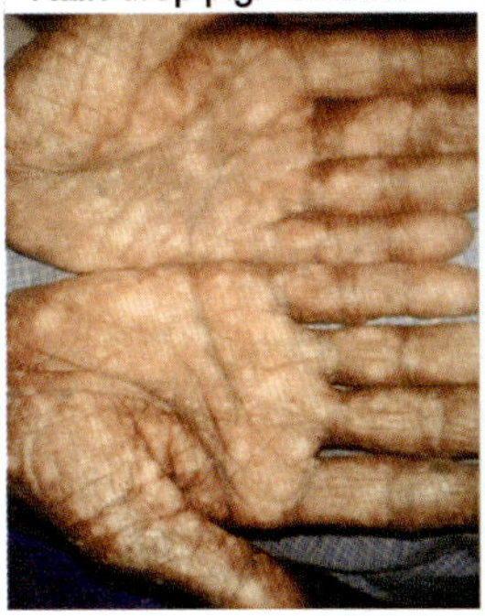

Hyperpigmented palms and soles

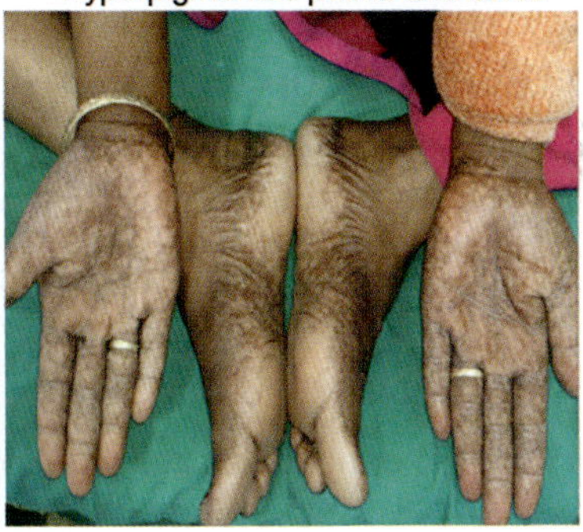

Other findings include:

- Red velvety stomach
- Subendocardial hemorrhage
- Flea bitten hemorrhage
- Glove and stocking peripheral neuropathy

7

CHAPTER

Pharmacology

1. MOA of vancomycin is:

A. Cell wall synthesis inhibition
B. Cell membrane inhibition
C. Peptide synthesis inhibition
D. 30s ribosome inhibition

ANS. **A**

Mechanism of action of cell wall synthesis inhibitors

- Beta lactam antibiotics: Transpeptidase blocker
- Vancomycin: Transglycosylation blocker
- Dephosphorylation blocker: Bacitracin
- Enol pyruvate transferase blocker: Fosfomycin
- Alanine ligase blocker: Cycloserine

Mechanism of action of protein synthesis inhibitors

- Aminoglycoside: Blocks initiation by binding to 30s
- Linezolid: Blocks initiation by binding to 50s
- Tetracycline: Blocks attachment of new amino acid to acceptor site
- Chloramphenicol: Peptidyltransferase blocker
- Macrolide, lincosamide, streptogramin: Blocks translocation

2. Which of the following drugs is to be immediately stopped in a patient of diabetes with HTN and serum creatinine level of 5.6 mg?

A. Metformin
B. Insulin
C. Metoprolol
D. Linagliptin

ANS. **A**

Metformin is contraindicated in patients with high creatinine because of the risk of lactic acidosis.

Specific side effects of OHA

Metformin

1. GI symptoms
2. B12 deficiency
3. Lactic acidosis (especially in patients with high creatinine, liver failure, alcoholism, cardiorespiratory insufficiency)

Pioglitazone

1. Unsafe in Renal failure, Liver failure, cardiac failure
2. Increased risk of bladder cancer
3. Osteoporosis

DPP-4 inhibitors

1. Upper respiratory tract infection
2. Renal toxicity (Vildagliptin is hepatotoxic)

(Safest DPP-4 inhibitor in renal failure is linagliptan)(asked in Nov AIIMS 2016 and May 2017)

SGLT2 inhibitors

1. UTI
2. Risk of bladder cancer

3. In a case of acute exacerbation of asthma, salbutamol was given and no improvement noticed, intravenous corticosteroids and aminophylline was given and condition improved. What is the mechanism of corticosteroid in acute asthma?

A. Corticosteroid increase bronchial responsiveness to salbutamol
B. Corticosteroids cause direct bronchodilation when used with xanthines
C. Corticosteroids indirectly increase the effect of xanthines on adenosine receptor
D. Corticosteroids increase mucociliary clearance.

ANS. **A**

Corticosteroids has a dual effect in acute asthma with an early facilitatory effect on airway beta 2 adrenoreceptor sensitivity and a later effect on airway inflammation, which further emphasizes the need for corticosteroids to be administered as early as possible during an acute asthma attack.

Newer monoclonal antibodies in respiratory condition

1. Pitakinra: IL-3 and 4 antagonist (used in bronchial asthma)
2. Resilizumab: IL-5 antagonist (used in bronchial asthma)
3. Mepolizumab: IL-5 blocker (useful in hypereisnophilic vasculitis)
4. Omalizumab: Against IG E (in bronchial asthma)
5. Pavilizumab: Used against respiratory syncitial virus **(AIIMS November 2016)**.

4. A patient presented with right lower quadrant pain. He was already treated for right renal stone disease. Which of the following opioid is partial agonist at MU and full agonist at Kappa?

A. Pentazocin B. Buprenorphine
C. Tramadol D. Fentanyl

ANS. **A**

Pentazocine: Partial agonist and antagonist at mu receptor, and agonist at kappa

Buprenorphine: Partial agonist at mu and antagonist at kappa

Tramadol: Affinity for mu is low, while that for kappa and delta is very low. (Tramadol also has an additional mechanism of inhibiting reuptake of NA and 5-HT, and thus activating monoaminergic spinal inhibition of pain. Its analgesic action is only partially reversed by opioid antagonist naloxone.

Fentanyl: Congener of pethidine, 80–100 times more potent than morphine. It is chemically unrelated to morphine, but interacts with opioid receptors and its actions are blocked by naloxone.

5. Which of the following is given in induction of anesthesia?

A. Lorazepam B. Bupivacaine
C. Neostigmine D. Dexmedetomidine

ANS. **A**

Intravenous inducing agents in anesthesia

1. Thiopentone sodium
2. Methohexitone sodium

3. Propafol
4. Etomidate
5. Benzodiazepines
6. Ketamine
7. Fentanyl

6. A placebo therapy given to one patient and new drug given to another patient. On comparing:

Heart rate in placebo (72), Drug (86)

SBP in placebo (110), Drug (150)

DBP in placebo (80), Drug (68)

Cardiac output in placebo (5), Drug (6)

A. Alpha 1 antagonist and Beta agonist
B. Alpha 1 agoinst and M3 agonist
C. Alpha 1 agonist and Beta agonist
D. Beta agonist and Beta 2 agonist

ANS. **A**

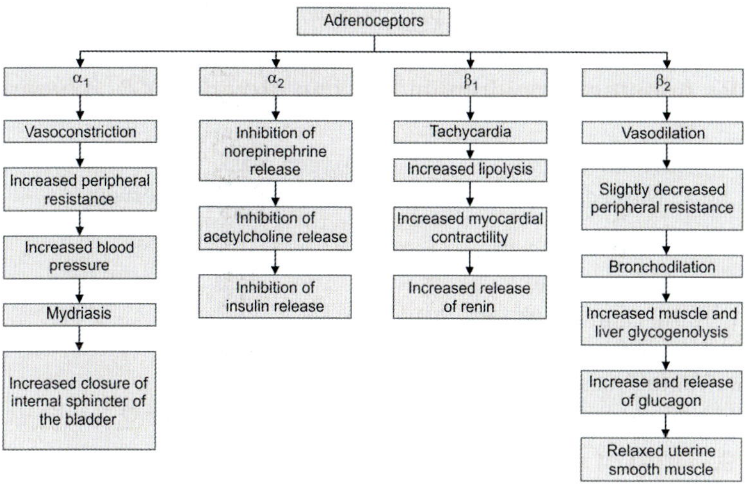

Alpha 1 produces increased peripheral resistance and increased diastolic pressure, hence the drug mentioned is alpha 1 antagonist.

Beta 1 produces tachycardia and increased systolic BP, hence drug is beta 1 agonist.

7. You have to give 180 mg of ceftriaxone to a patient in 2 mL syringe which has 10 divisions per mL. Concentration of this drug in vial is 500 mg/5 mL. How many divisions should be filled in 2 mL syringe to give 180 mg?

A. 18 B. 1.8
C. 2 D. 20

ANS. **A**

500 mg in 5 mL
So, 180 mg in $(180 \times 5)/500 = 1.8$ mL
Each 1 mL has 10 division so 1.8 mL has $1.8 \times 10 = 18$ divisions

Important formula in pharmacology

Volume of distribution = (dose administered /plasma conc) × body weight
Loading dose = (target plasma conc/bioavailablity) × volume of distribution
Maintenance dose = (target plasma conc./Bioavailablity) × clearance
T1/2 = (0.693 × volume of distribution/clearance)

8. Anesthetic equipment that can provide 100% oxygen is:

A. Venturi mask B. Oxygen mask
C. Nasal cannula D. Face mask with reservoir

ANS. **D**

Oxygen delivery by:
1. Nasal cannula: 24–44% FiO_2
2. Simple face mask: 40–60% FiO_2
3. Venturi mask: 24–40% FiO_2
4. Nonrebreathing mask (with reservoir bag): 60–100% O_2

9. Drug of choice for scrub typhus:

A. Doxycycline B. Azithromycin
C. Ciprofloxacin D. Chloramphenicol

ANS. **A**

Drug of choice for

Enterococci: Vancomycin
MRSA: Vancomycin
Acinetobacter: Meropenam
Brucella: Doxycycline and rifampicin

Enterobacter: Meropenem
Hemophilus influenza: Ceftriaxone
Pseudomonas: Piperacillin and tazobactam
Shigella: Ciprofloxacin
Vibrio: Tetracycline
Yersinia: Streptomycin
Melioidosis: Ceftazidime
Listeria: Ampicillin
Diphtheria: Erythromycin
Nocardia: Cotrimoxazole
Borrelia: Doxycycline
Chlamydia: Doxycycline
Rickettsiae: Doxycycline

10. Which of the following is not used in the emergency management of hyperkalemia?

A. Ca gluconate
B. IV $MgSO_4$
C. Insulin
D. Salbutamol nebulization

ANS. **B**

Treatment of hyperkalemia

1. If ECG changes are there, 10 mL 10% calcium gluconate slow IV over 10 minutes
   Action starts within 1 minute, lasts for 30 minutes
   MOA of calcium gluconate: Stabilizes myocardium
2. Insulin 10 units IV with dextrose 50 mL, 50%
3. Salbutamol nebulization 10 mg
4. Newer K+ binders: Sodium polystyrene sulfonate
5. Newer oral drug for hyperkalemia: Platiromer acetate

11. During resuscitation of septic shock, epinephrine was given to the patient. Its response is checked by seeing:

A. Increased HR
B. Decreased HR
C. Increased MAP
D. Decreased renal perfusion and reduced urine output

ANS. **C**

12. A diabetic, obese patient on metformin presents with uncontrolled sugar level even after increasing dosage. He is allergic to sulfonylureas, has pancreatitis and family history of bladder cancer.

He does not want to take injections, so what will you give next?

A. Sitagliptin
B. Liragliptide
C. Pioglitazone
D. Canagliflozin

ANS. **D**

Ruling out the options,
Liraglutide is a GLP 1 agonist, it is given via SC route.
Sitagliptin is contraindicated in pancreatitis
Pioglitazone has increased risk of bladder cancer.

13. Which one is a placebo?

A. Herbal medication with no effect known
B. Physiotherapy
C. Sham surgery
D. CBT

ANS. **C**

Sham surgery (placebo surgery) is a faked surgical intervention that omits the steps thought to be therapeutically necessary. In clinical trials of surgical interventions, Sham surgery is an important scientific control. This is because it isolates the specific effects of the treatment as opposed to the incidental effects caused by anesthesia, the incisional trauma, pre and postoperative care, and the patient's perception of having had a regular operation. The Sham surgery serves as an analogue to placebo drugs, neutralizing biases.

14. Drug of choice for gonococcal plus nongonococcal cervicitis:

A. Azithromycin 2 g oral single dose
B. Ciprofloxacin 500 mg oral single dose
C. Ceftriaxone 250 mg IM single dose
D. Cefixime 400 mg oral single dose

ANS. **A**

Nongonococcal urethritis is mainly caused by:

- *Chlamydia, Ureaplasma urealyticum, Mycoplasma, Haemophilus vaginalis*
- Now looking at options, cephalosporins are not active against mycoplasma species (lack of cell wall), hence ceftriaxone and cefixime are ruled out.
- Ciprofloxacin is also not active against mycoplasma, hence the correct answer is azithromycin.

15. A 27-year-old female came for treatment of infertility to OPD; bromocriptine was prescribed. What could be the possible reason?

A. Hyperprolactinemia
B. PCOD
C. Hypogonadotropic hypogonadism
D. PID

ANS. **A**

Uses of bromocriptine

1. Hyperprolactinemia
2. Acromegaly
3. Parkinsonism
4. Hepatic coma

16. What will you give in anaphylactic shock?

A. Adrenaline 0.5 mg 1/1000 IM
B. Adrenaline 1 mg 1/10000 IV
C. Atropine 3 mg
D. Adenosine 6 mg followed by 12 mg IV

ANS. **B**

Adrenaline is the drug of choice in anaphylactic shock. So options C and D are ruled out. Anaphylactic shock is a medical emergency. So we need to give drug so that it produces rapid action. Hence in anaphylactic shock, IV is preferred.

17. Treatment for motion sickness for a trip next morning?

A. Scopalamine patch a night before
B. Tab. Ranitidine one night before and then before the trip
C. Dimenhydrinate 1 hour before
D. Omeprazole

ANS. **A**

For the prophylaxis of motion sickness, apply scopalamine one patch behind ear at least 4–12 hours (preferably 12 hour) before anticipated exposure to motion.

18. Biofilm mechanism of resistance to antibiotics all, *except*:

A. Mechanical barrier
B. Increased excretion of antibiotics

C. Slow metabolism
D. Adherence

ANS. **D**

Bacteria that attach to a surface and grow as a biofilm are protected from killing by antibiotics. Reduced antibiotic susceptibility contributes to the persistence of biofilm infections such as those associated with implanted devices. The protective mechanisms at work in biofilms appear to be distinct from those that are responsible for conventional antibiotic resistance. In biofilms, poor antibiotic penetration, nutrient limitation and slow growth, adaptive stress responses, and formation of persister cells are hypothesized to constitute a multilayered defense. Each gene and gene product contributing to this resistance may be a target for the development of new chemotherapeutic agents. Disabling biofilm resistance may enhance the ability of existing antibiotics to clear infections involving biofilms that are refractory to current treatments.

19. A patient in labor ward was given opioid analgesic. Which drug should be kept ready for emergency?

A. Naloxone
B. Lignocaine
C. Diphenhydramine
D. Fentanyl

ANS. **A**

Opioid antagonists

1. Naloxone
2. Natrexone
3. Nalmefene

Clinical uses of Naloxone

1. Drug of choice for morphine poisoning (0.4–0.8 mg IV every 2–3 min; max 10 mg)
2. To reverse the respiratory depression due to intraoperative use of opioids
3. Diagnosis of opioid dependence
4. Partially reverses alcohol intoxication

20. What instruction do you give to a mother who is lactating regarding intake of drug?

A. No advice as most of drug are not secreted into breast milk
B. Give longer half-life drugs
C. Tell the mother to feed when it is least efficacious

D. Lactate Just before she take the next dose, when the plasma concentration of drug would be least.

ANS. **D**

Plasma concentration of drug varies with time follows the graph as shown below. Certain drugs can be secreted in breast milk and therefore transferred to the infant. Care should be taken to decrease this to the minimum possible levels.

Least plasma concentration of the drug will be just before the next loading dose. Hence, the least chance for the drug to be concentrated in milk and thereby transferred to the infant would be at the time just before taking next dose. Hence advice mother to lactate just before taking next dosage of the drug.

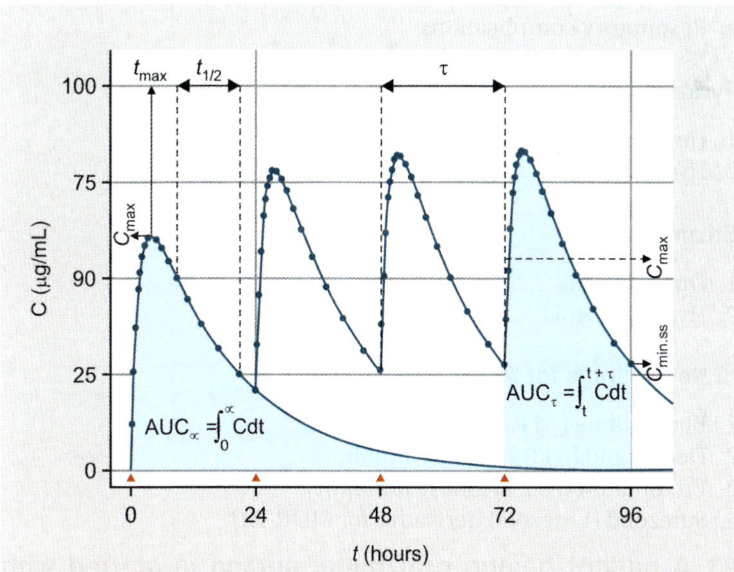

21. A patient in ATT develops tingling on lower limb. Which of the following drugs should be used?

A. Pyridoxine B. Thiamine
C. Folic acid D. B12

ANS. **A**

Specific side effect of ATT

INH

1. Hepatotoxicity

2. Pyridoxine deficiency
   (For prophylaxis—give10 mg/day and for treatment—give 100 mg/day)
3. Central nervous system (CNS) effects: Memory loss, psychosis, seizures
4. Systemic lupus erythematosus (SLE)
5. Shoulder hand syndrome
6. Cheese reaction

Rifampicin

1. Purpura
2. Hepatotoxicity
3. Orange colored urine
4. Respiratory complications

Pyrazinamide

1. Hepatotoxicity
2. Hyperuricemia

Ethambutol

1. Optic neuritis
2. Hyperuricemia

Newer drugs for MDR TB

1. Bedaquiline (ATP synthase inhibitor)
2. Delamanid (ATP synthase inhibitor)
3. Pretomanid (ATP synthase inhibitor)
4. Sutezolid (Linezolid derivative for MDR TB)

23. A patient having prinzmetal angina is started with ISMN. Patient got symptomatic relief from angina. What is the MOA?

A. Endothelium independent coronary vasodilatation
B. Reduced cardiac contractility
C. Increased left ventricular end diastolic volume
D. Decreased diastolic perfusion pressure

ANS. **A**

This is a direct question.

Important points on nitrates

1. All nitrates have high FPM metabolism except ISMN (Isosorbide mononitrate)
2. Skin rashes are maximum with Pentaerythritol tetranitrate
3. Nitrates used in acute attack: NTG and ISDN (Isosorbide dinitrite)

24. PSCK-9 inhibitor:

A. Alirocumab B. Mipomersan
C. Ezetimibe D. Lomitapide

ANS. **A**

Newer drugs for lipid lowering

1. PSCK-9 inhibitors
   - Alirocumab
   - Evolocumab
2. Mipomersan (inhibits apo B 100 synthesis)
3. Lopitamide [inhibits microsomal triglyceride transfer protein (MTP)]
   - Avasimibe (ACAT inhibitor)
   - Torcetrapib (CETP inhibitor)
   - Anacetrapib (CETP inhibitor)

25. Drug of choice for acute rejection after transplant:

A. Daclizumab B. Omalizumab
C. Cyclosporine D. Tacrolimus

ANS. **A**

26. New drug for breast cancer targeted against CDK4 and 6:

A. Safinamide B. Abemaciclib
C. Ocrelizumab D. Valbenazine

ANS. **B**

Newer drugs (asked in JIPMER nov 2017 session also)

1. Avelumab: AntiPD1 (programmed death ligand) approved for Merkel cell carcinoma
2. Dupulimab: Anti IL-4 receptor alpha for atopic dermatitis
3. Brodalimumab: Anti IL-17 receptor antibody for plaque psoriasis
4. Plecanatide/linaclotide: Guanylate cyclase C stimulator approved for treatment of chronic idiopathic constipation. It increases

CGMP, which stimulates CFTER, which increase CL-secretion into gut.

4. Naldemedine: Opioid antagonist for opioid induced constipation
5. Telotrisat: Tryptophan hydroxylase inhibitor for carcinoid syndrome
6. Midostaurin: Multikinase inhibitor approved for AML
7. Ocrelizumab: Anti CD 20 antibody for multiple sclerosis
8. Abolaparatide: PTH analogue for high-risk fracture
9. Valbenazine: VMAT 2 inhibitor for tardive dyskinesia
10. Safinamide: MAO B inhibitor for on-off phenomenon in parkinsonism
11. Abemaciclib/rivociclib/palbociclib: CDK 4 and 6 inhibitor for ER + postmenopausal breast cancer
12. Niraparib: PARP (poly ADP-ribose polymerase) inhibitor for ovarian, fallopian and primary peritoneal cancer resistant of cisplatin.
13. Lesinurad: Used in gout
14. Sarilumab: Anti IL-6 for rheumatoid arthritis.

8
CHAPTER

Obstetrics and Gynecology

1. Identify the grip in the picture used for checking ballotability of head:

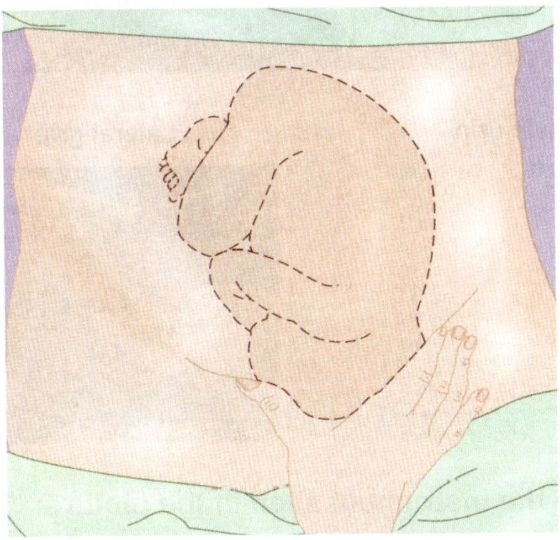

A. Pelvic grip B. Pawlick grip
C. Fundal grip D. Umblical grip

ANS. **B**

Importance of Pawlick's grip: To determine which part of fetus occupies the lower part of uterus.

Grips

Fundal grip

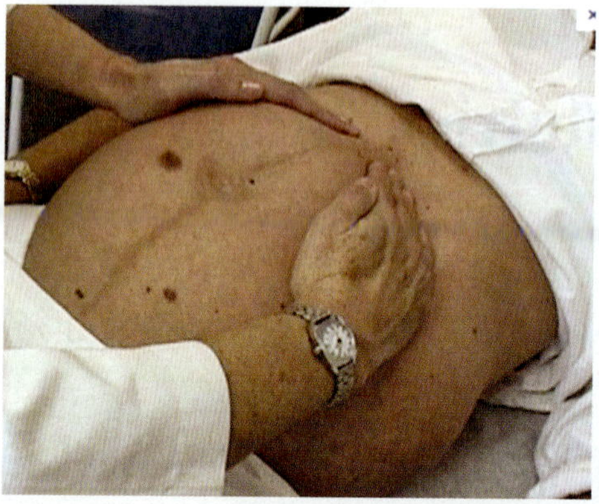

Second pelvic grip

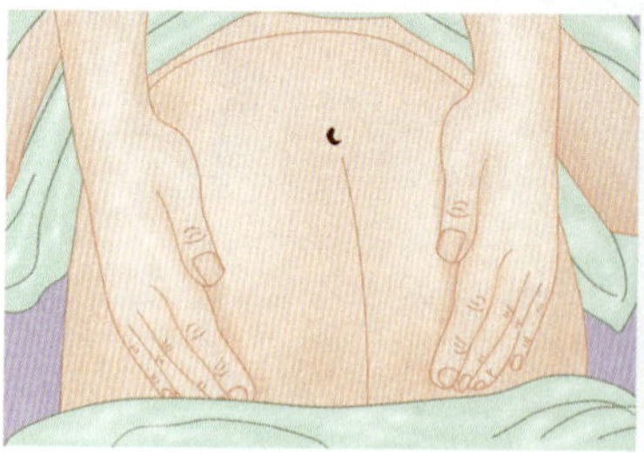

Lateral grip

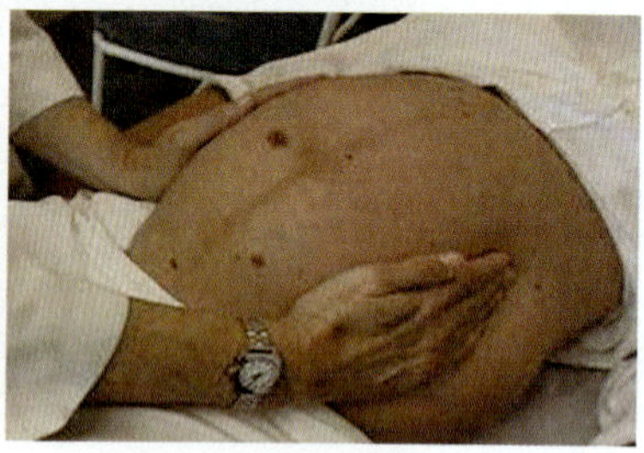

2. Name the instrument seen in the picture:

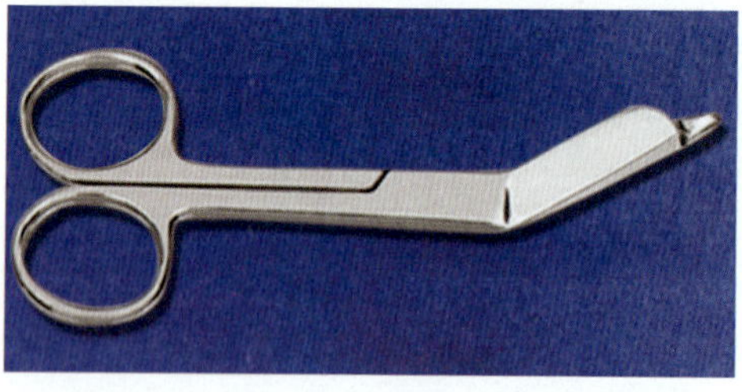

A. Mayo scissor
B. Episiotomy scissor
C. Dressing scissors
D. Cervical scissor

ANS. **C**

Episiotomy scissor: Angulated scissor used to prevent extension of pelvic tear into the anal margins.

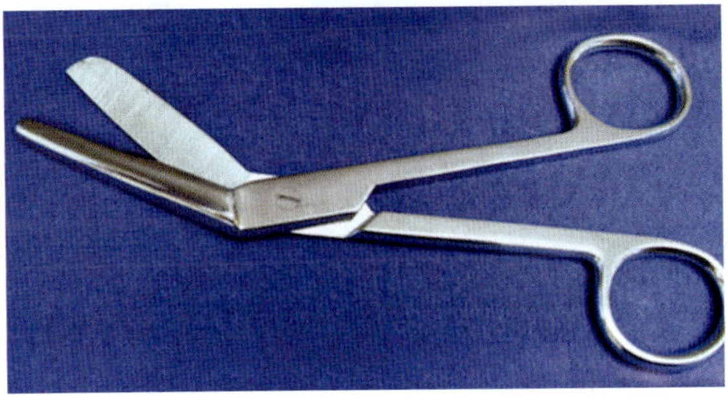

Structures cut in episiotomy:
1. Plain and subcutaneous tissue.
2. Vaginal mucosa.
3. Superficial and deep transverse perineil, bulbospongiosus, levator ani.
4. Internal pundendal vessels.

Degrees of perineal tear:
1. 1st degree: Only perineal skin is cut.
2. 2nd degree: Perineal muscles (episiotomy).
3. 3rd degree:
   - 3a: <50% of exterior sphincter
   - 3b: >50% of exterior sphincter
   - 3c: Internal sphincter
4. 4th degree: Rectal mucosa.

Other instruments that can be asked

Ovum forceps

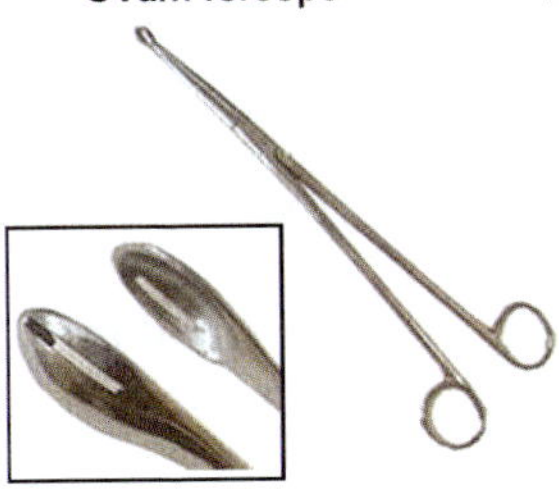

Babcock's forceps

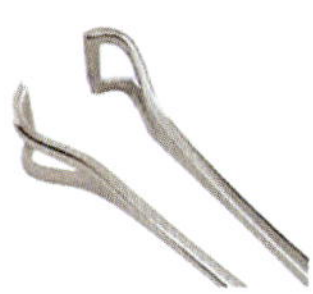

Doyen's retractor

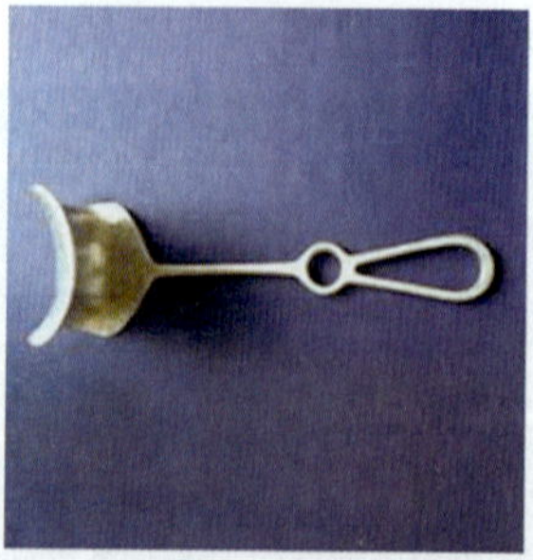

Deaver's retractor

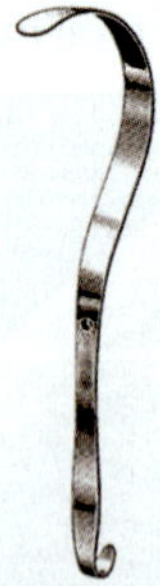

3. In partogram, time of initial markings are made in:

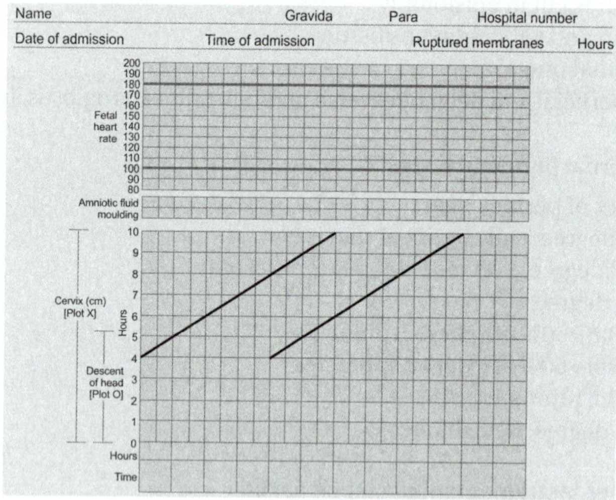

A. Left of alert line
B. Left of action line
C. Right of alert line
D. Right of action line

ANS. **A**

Modified World Health organization partogram:
1. Latent phase removed.
2. Active phase begins from 4 cm cervical dilatation.
3. 4 hours difference between alert of action time.

Another important topic with regard to partogram is arrest labor (AIIMS November 2016)

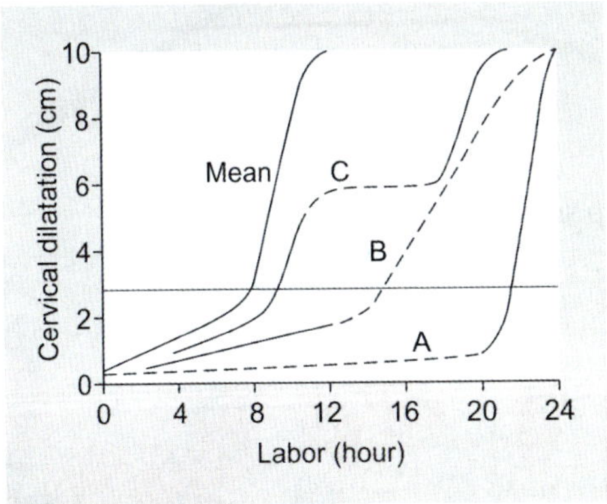

A: Prolonged latent phase
B: Prolonged active phase
C: Arrest in active phase (secondary arrest).

Arrest of active phase

No change in cervical dilatation for more than 4 hours.

Arrest of second stage arrest

- No descend of head in primigravida for 3 hours and multigravida for 2 hours
- Treatment of arrest: CS.

4. Nanovalent vaccine offers protection against which type of HPV viruses?

A. 6, 8, 10, 11, 31, 33, 45, 52, 58
B. 6, 11, 16, 18, 31, 33, 45, 52, 58
C. 6, 11, 16, 18, 31, 35, 45, 52, 58
D. 6, 11, 16, 18, 31, 32, 33, 34

ANS. **B**

HPV vaccine:
- Cervarix: Bivalent—16 and 18
- Gardasil: Quadrivalent: 6, 11, 16 and 18
- Nanovalent vaccine: 6, 11, 16, 18, 31, 33, 45, 52, 58
- 3 doses: 0, 2, and 6 months
- 0.5 mL given IM.

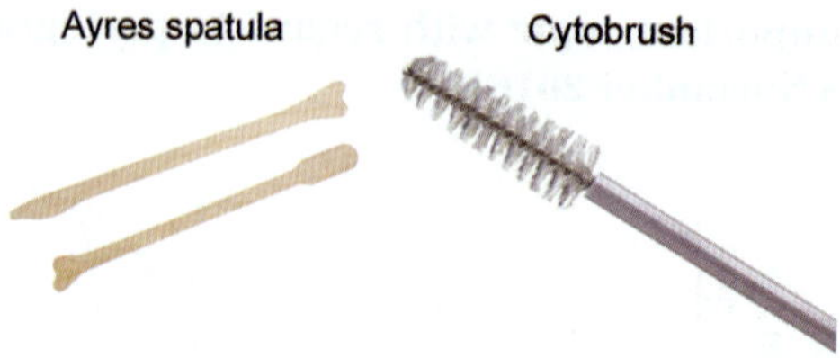

Images in Pap smear

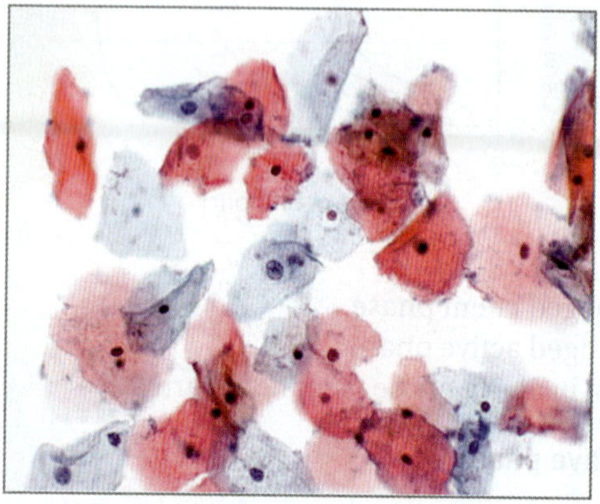

Three types of cells in Pap smear:

1. Superficial: Red cells—estrogen dependent
2. Intermediate: Greenish-blue—progesterone dependent
3. Parabasal: Blue—does not respond to estrogen/progesterone

Important points in Pap smear:

1. In menopause, there is excess parabasal cells.
2. Basal cells never occur in Pap smear, if present it indicates erosion.

5. According to Naegele's rule, calculate EDD of a patient with LMP 9/1/2017:

A. 16/10/2017 B. 16/09/2017
C. 16/11/2017 D. 09/10/2017

ANS. **A**

- Adding 7 days + 9 months to LMP gives EDD
- Naegele's rule is based on 28 days regular cycle
- If the cycle is shorter or longer than 28 days, EDD will be corrected and written as corrected EDD.

For irregular cycles:

1. If she is having 40 days cycle regularly, to get corrected EDD, add (40–28) with the EDD calculated from LMP.

2. If she is having 21 days cycle regularly, to get corrected EDD, substract (28–21) 7 with the EDD calculated from LMP.

6. A primigravida came with 6 cm cervical dilatation with contraction rate of 3/10 minutes. Which stage of labor is she in?

A. 1st stage
B. 2nd stage
C. 3rd stage
D. 4th stage

ANS. **A**

- 1st stage (onset of true labor pain to full cervical dilatation)
- 2nd stage (delivery of baby)
- 3rd stage (delivery of placenta
- 4th stage (1 hour observation).

Pictorial representation of stages of labor

Stages of labor

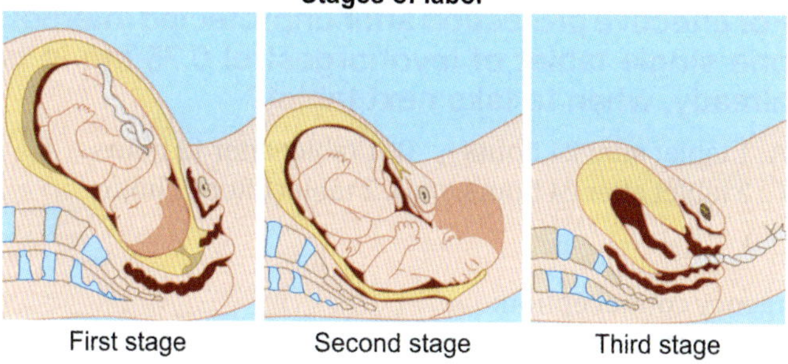

7. Post-menopausal female with biopsy report as endometrial hyperplasia with atypia. Next line of management is:

A. Type 1 hysterectomy
B. Oral progestins
C. Mirena
D. Dilatation and curettage

ANS. **A**

Types of endometrial hyperplasia:
1. Simple
2. Complex

Causes of hyperplasia:
1. PCOD
2. Follicular cyst
3. Granulosa and theca cell tumor
4. Hormone replacement therapy.

Chances of malignancy

1. Simple hyperplasia without atypia: 1%.
2. Simple hyperplasia with atypia: 8%.
3. Complex hyperplasia without atypia: 3%.
4. Complex hyperplasia with atypia: 29%.

Treatment of hyperplasia with atypia

1. For postmenopausal type 1/simple hysterectomy
2. Young women, not completed family—progesterone (medroxy progesterone acetate) levonorgestrel-releasing intrauterine system (LNG-IUS) + biopsy 3 monthly.

Treatment of hyperplasia without atypia

Progesterone (medroxy progesterone acetate) LNG-IUS + biopsy 3 monthly.

8. For effective protection after unprotected intercourse, one single tablet of levonorgestrel 0.75 mg is taken already, when to take next tablet?

A. 1 tablet after 24 hours
B. 1 tablet after 12 hours
C. 2 tablet after 24 hours
D. 2 tablet after 12 hours

ANS. **B**

Emergency contraception:

1. Yuzpe method (within 72 hours: High dose OCP 2 + 2 (12 hours apart) or low dose OCP 4 + 4 (12 hours apart).
2. LNG 0.75 mg 1 tab immediately, 2nd tab after 12 hours.
3. Mifepristone (RU 486).
4. Ulipristal 30 mg tab—5 days.
5. Copper-T IUD

Images of copper containing IUD

CU-T380A

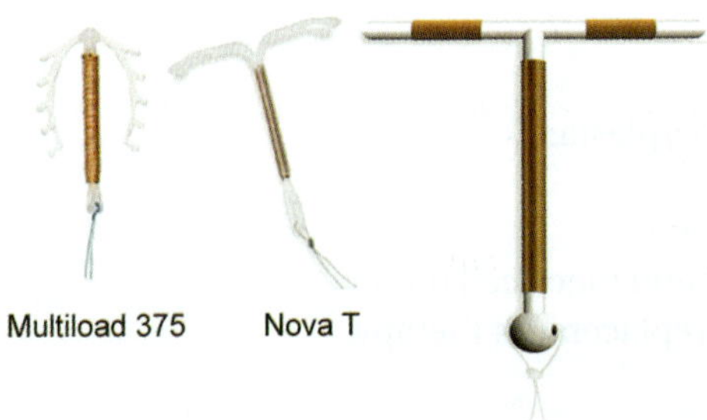

Image of Mirena (total LNG is 52 mg and is released at a rate of 20 μg/day for a period of 5 years)

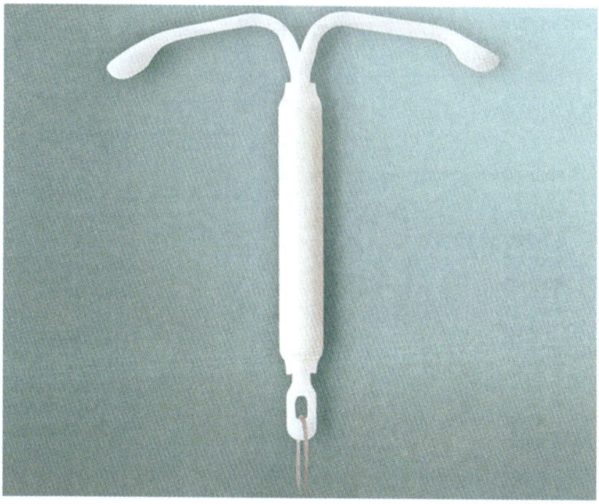

9. Father of 2 children, now they are not able to conceive is diagnosed to have hypogonadotropic hypogonadism, which of the following is not true?

A. Low luteinizing hormone (LH) and follicle-stimulating hormone (FSH)
B. Low testosterone
C. Oligospermia
D. High prolactin levels

ANS. **D**

- Hypogonadotropic hypogonadism: Low LH and FSH, low testosterone, azoospermia, low prolactin level
- Hypergonadotropic hypogonadism: High LH and FSH, low testosterone, azoospermia, high prolactin level.
- Normogonadotropic: Normal, LH, FSH, Testosterone— azoospermia.

10. 18-year-old girl with primary amenorrhea having a karyotype of 45X0 presents with infantile uterus. What should be done next?

A. Hormone replacement therapy (HRT) to induce pubertyB. Vaginoplasty
C. Clitoroplasty
D. Bilateral gonadectomy

ANS. **A**

Here the diagnosis is Turner's syndrome.

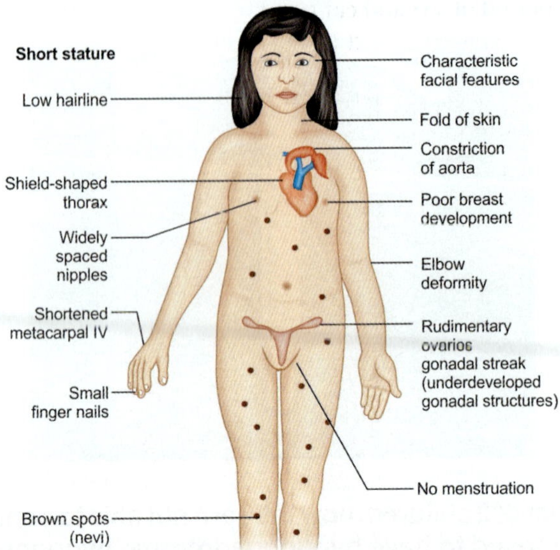

The primary treatments for all girls and women with Turner's syndrome include hormone therapies (growth hormone and estrogen).

It is important to identify a Y chromosome because affected individuals are at a risk of gonadoblastoma (20 to 30%). Only in such cases we need to do gonadectomy.

Hence, the answer for this question is HRT to induce Puberty.

Evaluation of primary amenorrhea

Secondary sexual characters

Normal
- MRKH
- AIS
- Transverse vaginal septum
- Imperforate hymen

Absent
- Turner's syndrome
- Kallman syndrome
- Swyer's syndrome

Abbreviation: MRKH, Mayer-Rokitansky-Küster-Hauser; AIS, Androgen insensitivity syndrome

11. A primigravida was given dietary advice in the 2nd trimester. What should be the extra calorie intake in pregnancy?

A. 200 kcal
B. 300 kcal
C. 500 kcal
D. No extra calorie

ANS. **B**

- In pregnancy: Add 350 kcal of energy and 23 g protein
- For lactation: Add 600 kcal of energy (up to 6 months) and 520 kCal (after 6 months) and 19 g protein.

Normal changes in pregnancy	
Hematological changes	*Cardiovascular changes*
Plasma volume increases by 40%	Cardiac output increases by 40%
Red cell volume increases by 20%	Pulse rate increases by 10% or 15 bpm
Physiological dilution in pregnancy	Stroke volume increases by 10%
Hemoglobin and hematocrit decrease	Peripheral vascular resistance falls
WBC count increases	Mean arterial pressure and DBP falls
Platelets normal or slight decrease by 15%	Colloid oncotic pressure falls
Total proteins increase	
Plasma protein concentration decreases	
Albumin decreases	
Globulins increase slightly	
Albumin: globulin decrease 1:1	
Fibrinogen increases by 50%	
Increase in factor VIII, IX and X	*Renal changes*
Decrease in anticoagulants	Renal blood flow increases by 80%
Inhibition of fibrinolytic activity	GFR increases by 50%
ESR increases four times	Creatinine and other clearances increased
Serum iron decreases	Serum creatinine, urea and urate decreased
Total iron binding capacity increases	Glycosuria may be normal

Abbreviations: WBC, white blood cell; GFR, glomerular filtration rate; ESR, erythrocyte sedimentation rate; DBP, diastolic blood pressure

Parameters which does not change in pregnancy?

1. pH
2. Vital capacity
3. FEV1

4. Inspiratory reserve volume
5. Pulmonary capillary wedge pressure
6. Respiratory rate.

12. You treat a 27-year-old infertile patient with bromocriptine. What should be the diagnosis?

A. Hyperpituitarism
B. Hypopituitarism
C. Polycystic ovarian disease (PCOD)
D. Hyperprolactinemia

ANS. **D**

Clinical manifestations of hyperprolactinemia	
Women	*Men*
• Galactorrhea 30–80% • Menstrual irregularity • Infertility	• Galactorrhea <30% • Impotence

Other manifestations

- Visual field abnormalities
- Headaches
- Extraocular muscle weakness
- Anterior pituitary malfunction

Hypogonadism in both women and men by suppressing gonadotropin-releasing hormone (GnRh) secretion and pulsatility, resulting in low level of LH and FSH.

Medical therapeutic options for the management of hyperprolactinemia

- Dopamine agonists are currently the first therapeutic option
- Dopamine agonists have proven efficacy in reducing prolactin levels, restoring ovulation in premenopausal women and restoring gonadal function in men
- Bromocriptine has been used the longest
- Cabergoline has greater affinity and selectivity for pituitary dopamine D2 receptor and longer duration of action.

13. 35-year-old woman comes with post-coital bleeding, What is the next step?

A. Pap smear
B. Conization
C. Cryotherapy
D. Targeted biopsy

ANS. **A**

- Answer is Pap smear, because they have asked for the next diagnosis
- The best diagnosis is always colposcopy-guided biopsy.

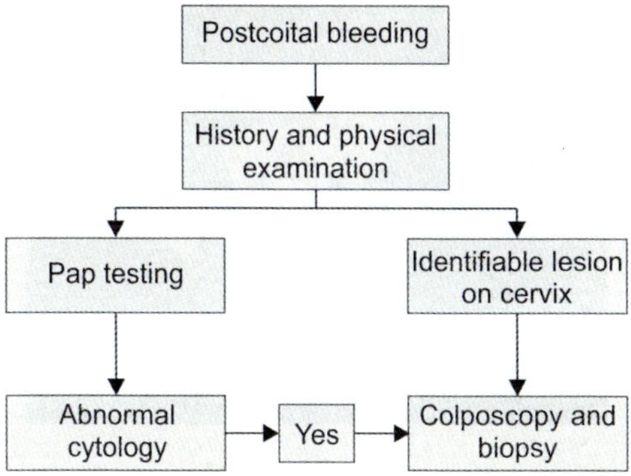

Other important topics in obstetrics

HSG images

Tuberculosis of the fallopian tube (golf club appearance on HSG)

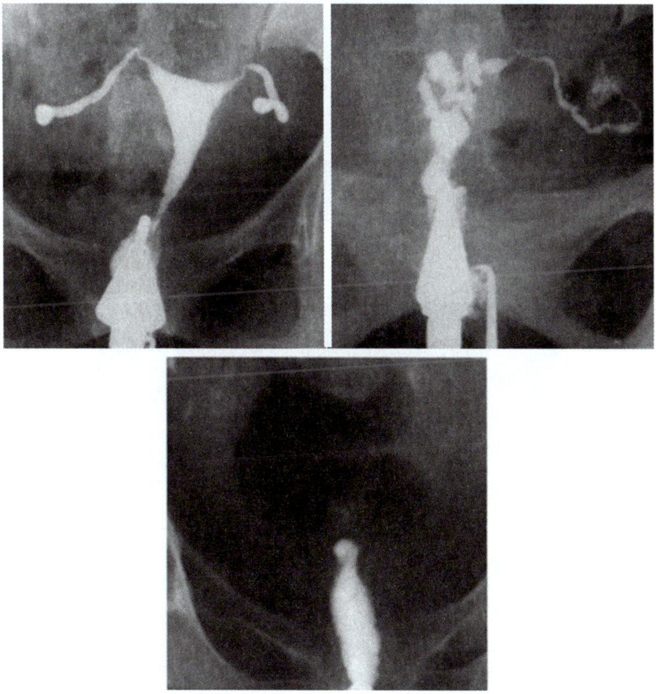

Asherman's syndrome

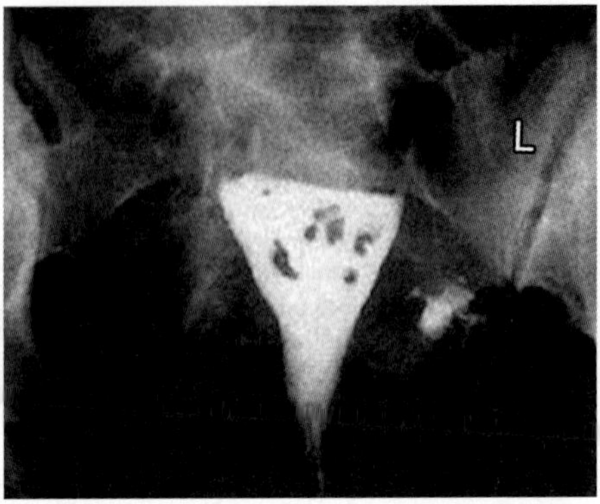

Uterine didelphys

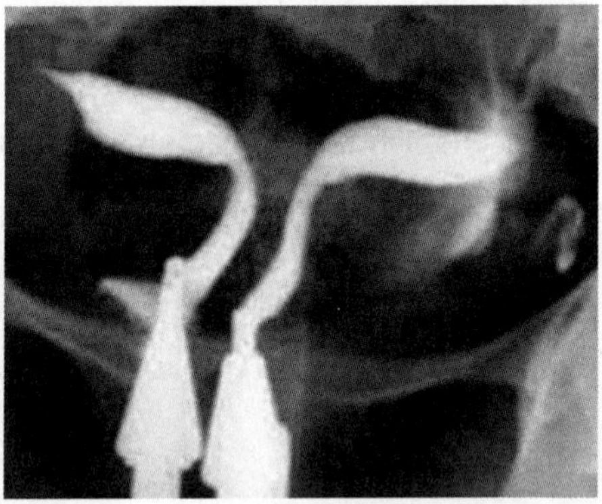

Septate uterus

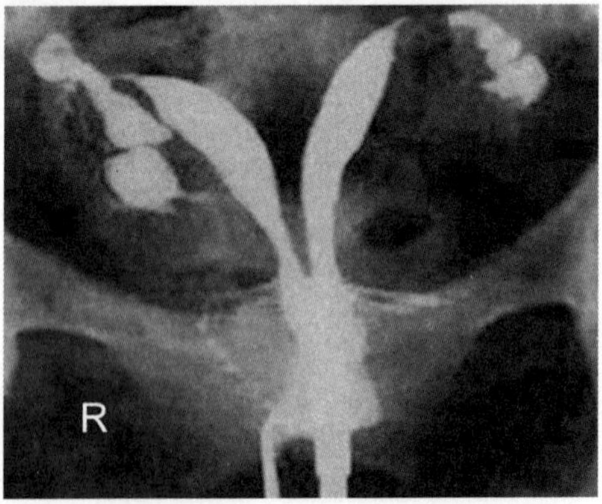

Bicornuate uterus

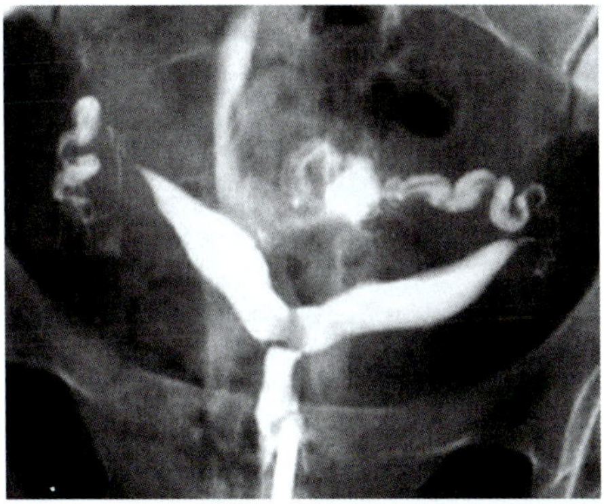

Histology of secretory phase of menstrual cycle

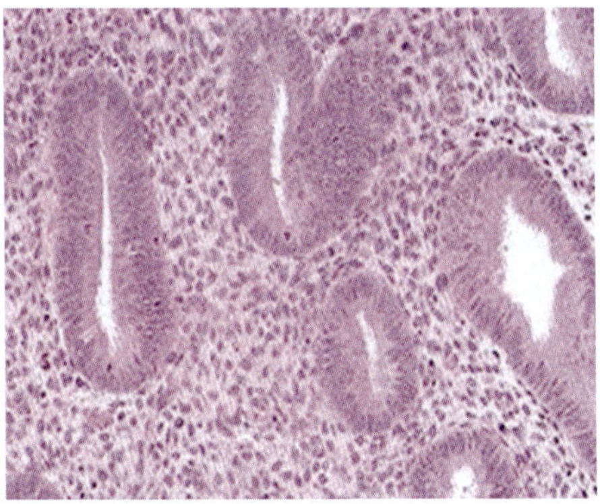

Histology of proliferative phase (subnuclear vacuolation)

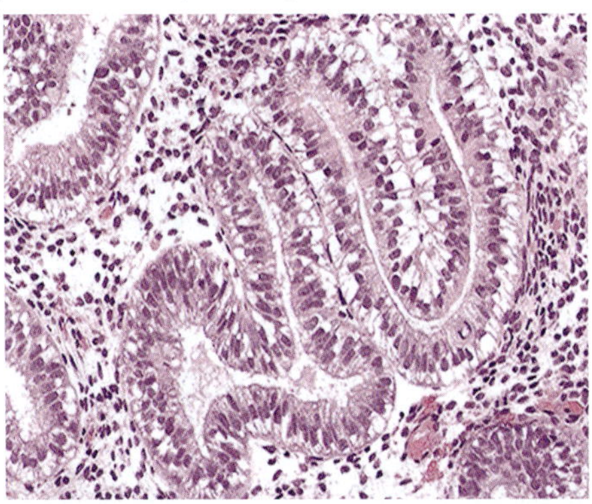

Important USG images

Snowstorm appearance (hydatiform mole)

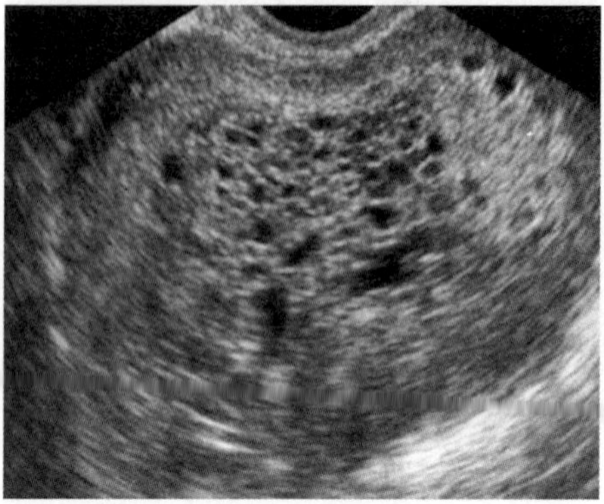

Ovarian hyperstimulation syndrome (OHSS)

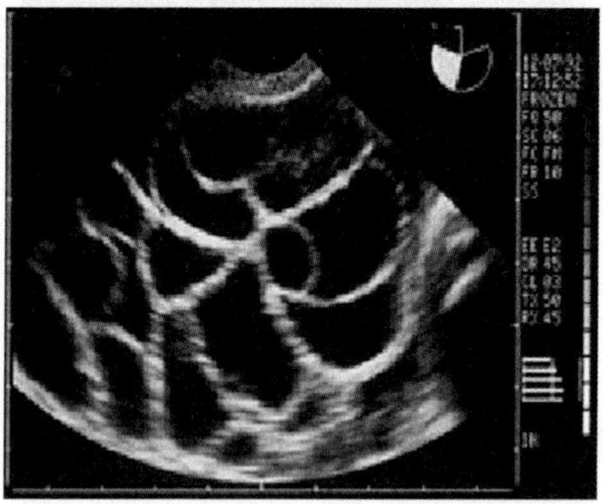

Polycystic Ovary Syndrome

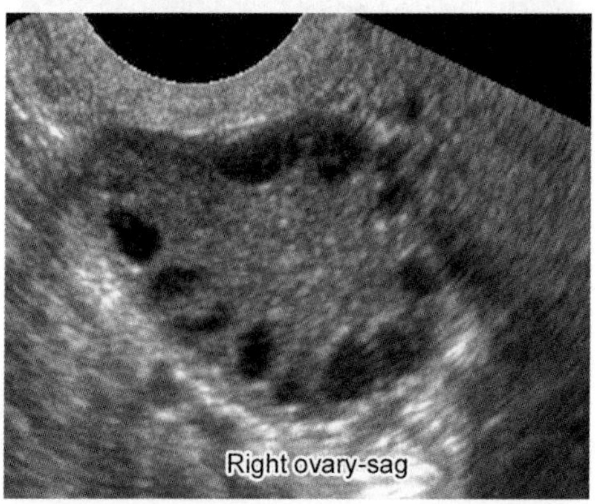

Nuchal translucency

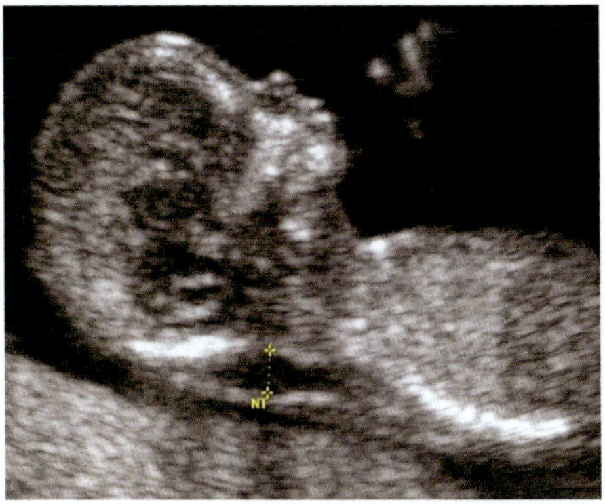

Cystic hygroma

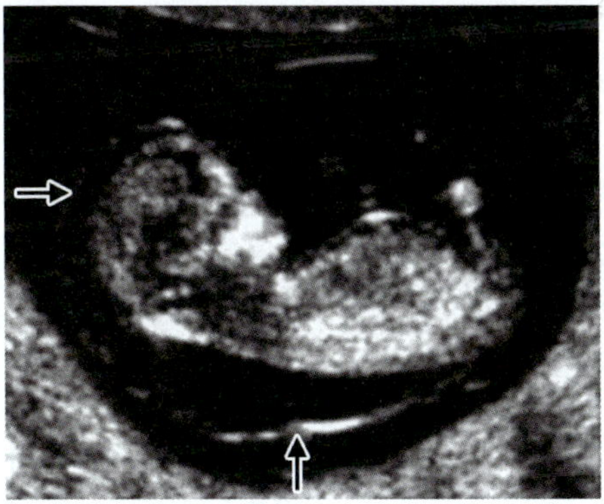

Rokitansky protuberance (dermoid)

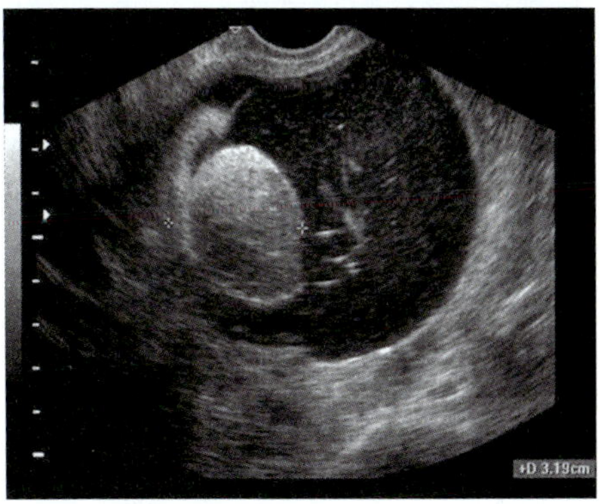

CTG images (cardiotocography images)

Late deceleration seen in uteroplacental insufficiency

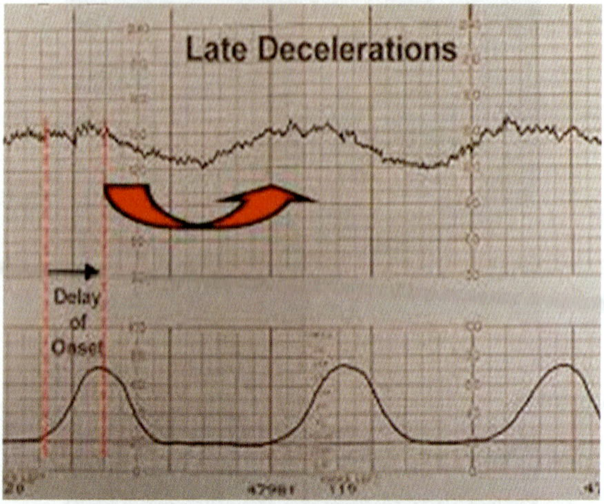

Early deceleration in head compression

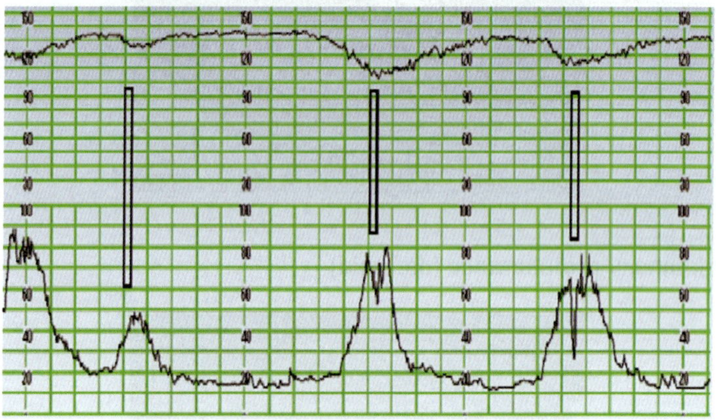

Variable deceleration in cord prolapse

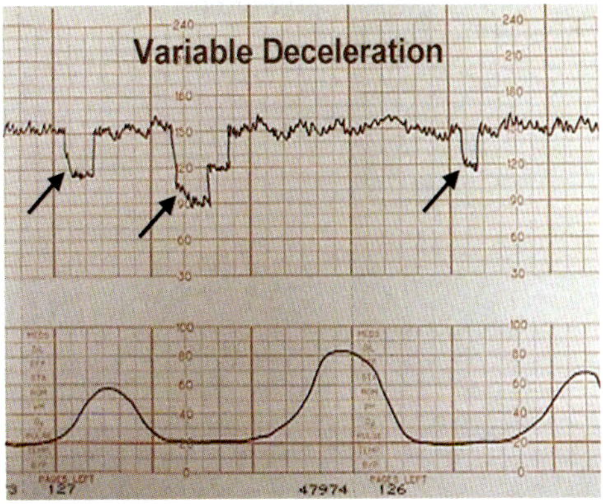

Sinusoidal pattern in anemia, hypoxia

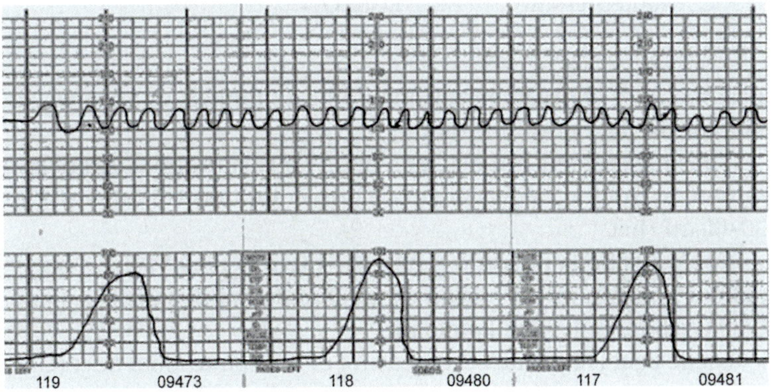

9 CHAPTER

Surgery

1. Best tool for monitoring the fluid resuscitation in trauma patients:

A. Urine output
B. Central venous pressure
C. Blood pressure
D. SPO_2

ANS. **A**

Best measure of organ perfusion and best monitor for adequacy of fluid resuscitation is urine output.

The only problem is that it is an hourly measure and does not give minute to minute value (Adequate urine output is 0.5 mL/kg/hr or 30–60 mL/hr).

Central venous pressure (CVP): As there is no CVP for a shock patient and cannot be placed as an assessment of shock as alone. CVP is a poor reflector of preload.

- Lactic acid is the one best measure of gastrointestinal tract (GIT) perfusion
- Consciousness is the best measure of brain perfusion.

2. Modified shock index formula is:

A. Heart rate/mean arterial pressure (MAP)
B. Heart rate/systolic blood pressure (SBP)
C. Heart rate/diastolic blood pressure (DBP)
D. BP/heart rate

ANS. **A**

- Shock index is heart rate/MAP
- Modified shock index = HR/MAP
- MAP = DBP + 1/3 × pulse pressure

Important scores in trauma

1. Revised trauma scale:
   Glasgow coma scale (GCS) + systolic BP + respiratory rate (RR)
2. TRISS—trauma score injury severity score
   Revised trauma score (RTS) + age + injury severity score
3. MESS—mangled extremity severity score:
   Age + limb ischemia + energy of impact + shock
4. EMTRAS—emergency trauma score:
   Age, GCS, prothrombin time (PT) + base excess

3. 22 gauge IV cannula color is:

A. Gray B. Blue
C. Pink D. Green

ANS. **B**

14 gauge means 14 needles kept side by side makes an inch

Gauge	*Color code*	*External diameter*	*Length*	*Flow rate*
14 G	Orange	2.1 mm	45 mm	240 mL/min
16 G	Gray	1.8 mm	45 mm	180 mL/min
18 G	Green	1.3 mm	32/45 mm	90 mL/min
20 G	Pink	1.1 mm	32 mm	60 mL/min
22 G	Blue	0.9 mm	25 mm	36 mL/min
24 G	Yellow	0.7 mm	19 mm	20 mL/min
26 G	Violet	0.6 mm	19 mm	13 mL/min

4. French in Foley's catheter refers to:

A. Diameter of catheter B. Outer circumference
C. Inner circumference D. Lumen size

ANS. **A**

French size in three times the diameter in millimeters. A round catheter of 1 French has an external diameter of 1/3 mm. Hence, diameter of round catheter in mm = French size/3.

Silicone catheter

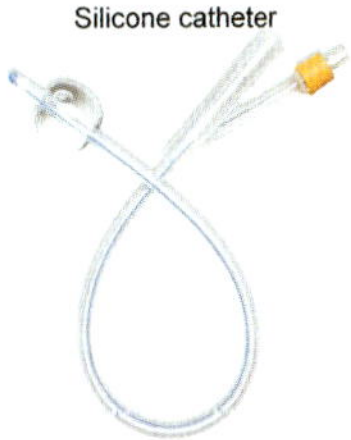

Malecot catheter

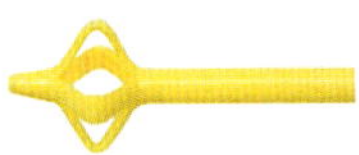

Swan ganz catheter

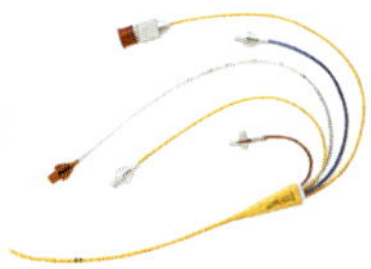

5. In a preoperative patient surgical checklist which of the following is not needed?

A. Oral consent B. Doctor signature
C. Site marking D. Confirming patient's identity

ANS. **B**

Surgical safety checklist: Sign in, time out, sign out

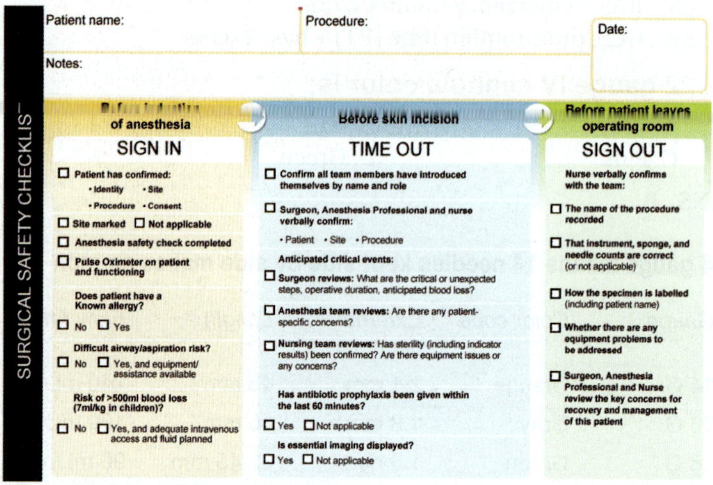
SURGICAL SAFETY CHECKLIST

Patient name: Procedure: Date:

Notes:

Before induction of anesthesia — SIGN IN

- ☐ Patient has confirmed: • Identity • Site • Procedure • Consent
- ☐ Site marked ☐ Not applicable
- ☐ Anesthesia safety check completed
- ☐ Pulse Oximeter on patient and functioning

Does patient have a Known allergy?
☐ No ☐ Yes

Difficult airway/aspiration risk?
☐ No ☐ Yes, and equipment/ assistance available

Risk of >500ml blood loss (7ml/kg in children)?
☐ No ☐ Yes, and adequate intravenous access and fluid planned

Before skin incision — TIME OUT

- ☐ Confirm all team members have introduced themselves by name and role
- ☐ Surgeon, Anesthesia Professional and nurse verbally confirm: • Patient • Site • Procedure

Anticipated critical events:

- ☐ Surgeon reviews: What are the critical or unexpected steps, operative duration, anticipated blood loss?
- ☐ Anesthesia team reviews: Are there any patient-specific concerns?
- ☐ Nursing team reviews: Has sterility (including indicator results) been confirmed? Are there equipment issues or any concerns?

Has antibiotic prophylaxis been given within the last 60 minutes?
☐ Yes ☐ Not applicable

Is essential imaging displayed?
☐ Yes ☐ Not applicable

Before patient leaves operating room — SIGN OUT

Nurse verbally confirms with the team:

- ☐ The name of the procedure recorded
- ☐ That instrument, sponge, and needle counts are correct (or not applicable)
- ☐ How the specimen is labelled (including patient name)
- ☐ Whether there are any equipment problems to be addressed
- ☐ Surgeon, Anesthesia Professional and Nurse review the key concerns for recovery and management of this patient

6. Which of the following is called balanced resuscitation?

A. Giving colloids and crystalloids at a ratio of 1:1
B. Maintaining pH ensuring acid-base balance
C. Maintaining permissible hypotension to avoid bleeding
D. Maintaining airway, breathing and circulation

ANS. **C**

Components of damage control resuscitation:

1. Permissive hypotension essential definitive surgical control
2. Minimize crystalloid use
3. Initial use of 5% hypertoxic saline
4. Early use of blood products
5. Treat coagulopathy

7. Identify the diagnosis of the given gross specimen?

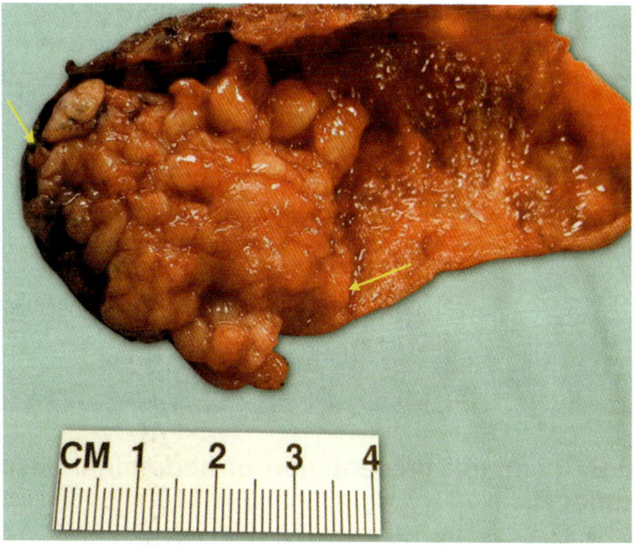

A. Carcinoma gallbladder
B. Gallbladder polyp
C. Cholesterosis
D. Adenomyomatosis gallbladder

ANS. **B**

Cholesterosis (Strawberry gallbladder)

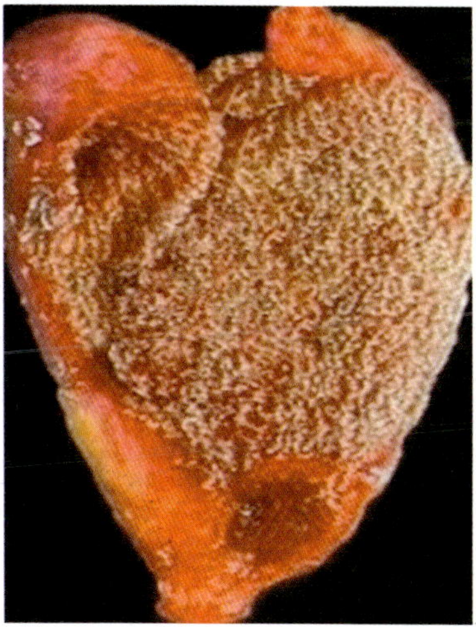

Adenomyomatosis gallbladder

USG shows comet tail artefact

MRI shows pearl of necklace pattern

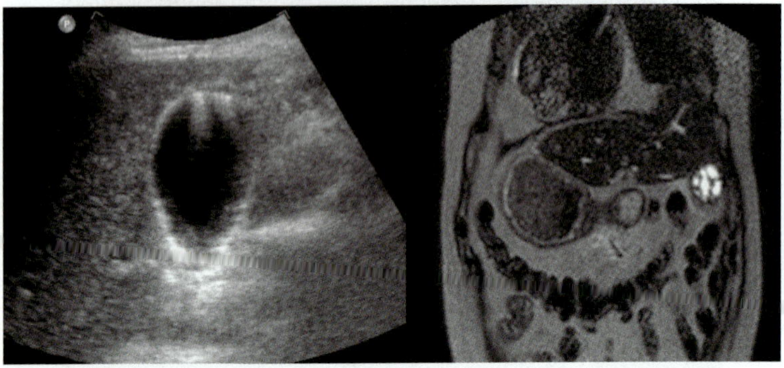

8. Most common presentation of abdominal desmoid tumor is:

A. Abdominal pain B. Abdominal mass
C. Fever D. Rectal prolapse

ANS. **B**

Desmoid tumor

- Presents as painless abdominal mass
- Associated with familial adenomatous polyposis (FAP) and Gardner's syndrome
- Locally invasive, hence treated with excision and adjuvant radiotherapy (RT).

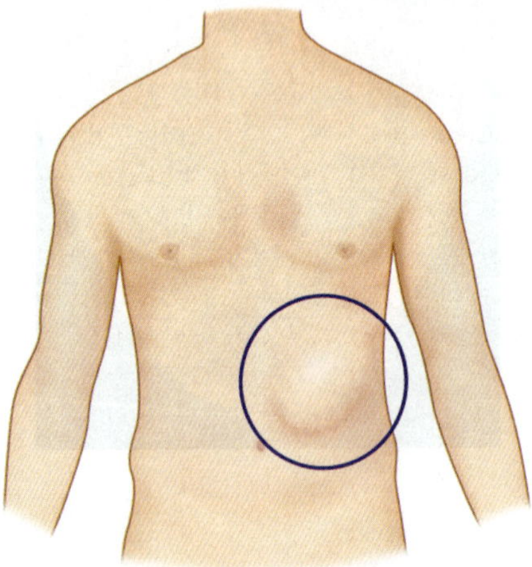

CT of a desmoid tumor

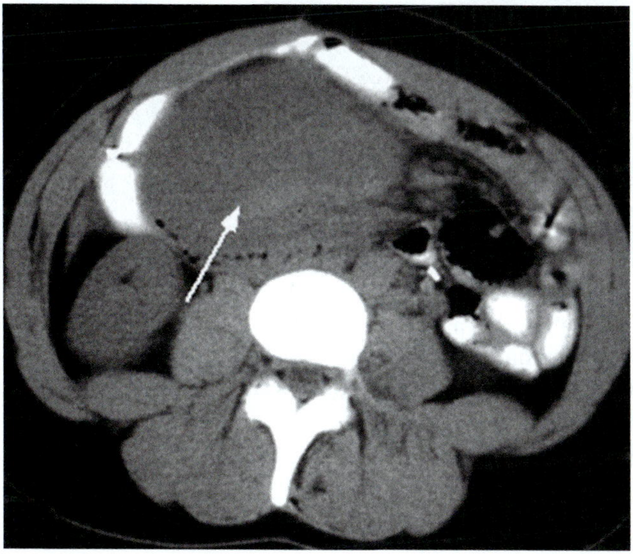

9. A 10-year-old child with pain and mass in right lumbar region with no fever, with right hip flexed and X-ray shows spine changes. Most probable diagnosis is:

A. Psoas abscess
B. Pyonephrosis
C. Retrocecal appendicitis
D. Torsion of right undescended testes

ANS. **A**

Psoas abscess

An abscess in the psoas muscle of the abdomen may be caused by lumbar tuberculosis. Owing to the proximal attachments of the iliopsoas, such an abscess may drain inferiorly into the upper medial thigh and present as a swelling in the region. The sheath of the muscle arises from the lumbar vertebrae and the intervertebral discs between the vertebrae. The disc is more susceptible to infection, from tuberculosis and *Salmonella discitis*. The infection can spread into the psoas muscle sheath.

Treatment may involve drainage and antibiotics

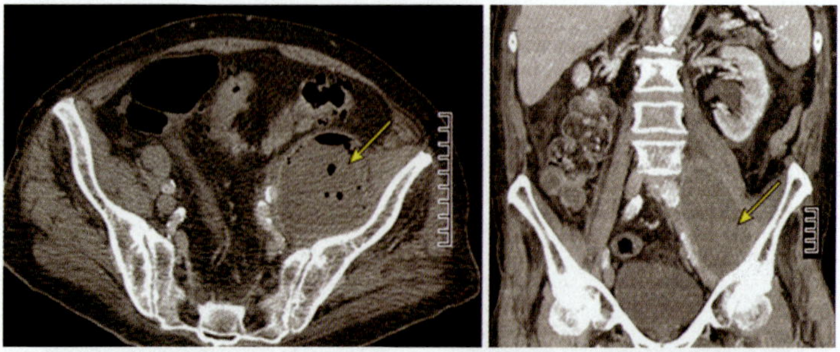

10. How will you check the functioning of the ICD tube?

A. By seeing for continuous air bubbles coming out of the drain
B. By seeing the movement of air water column during respiration
C. By chest X-ray
D. Auscultation

ANS. **B**

- The functioning of the tube can be confirmed by seeing the column of water in the chest tube moving up and down during respiration.
- If underwater drainage tube fails to expand a lung of open pneumothorax, we use 5 cm water low pressure suction.
- Heimlich valve is a special valve used instead of underwater drain only for pneumothorax cases.

The three bottle suction system for chest drainage

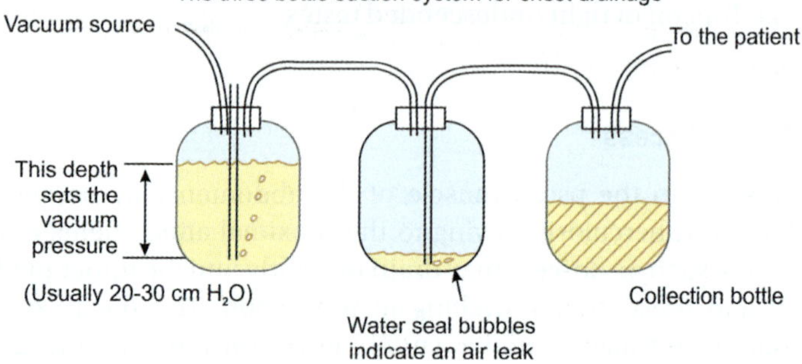

Heimlich valve

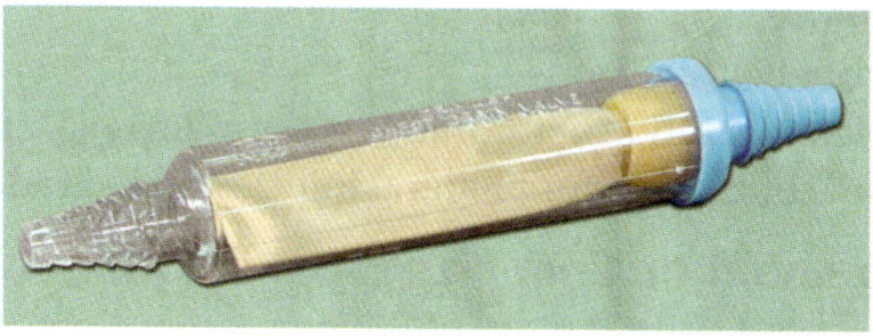

11. Following a blunt trauma abdomen—a patient had renal laceration and urinoma. Even after 12 days, urinoma persisted, but patient was stable, no fever, what will you do next?

A. Percutaneous nephrostomy
B. J-shaped urinary stent
C. Wait and watch
D. Explore

ANS. **B**

In this question both Wait and Watch and ureteric stenting is possible. But better answer would be ureteric stenting as a persisting urinoma can lead to ureter blockade and hydronephrosis.

Small amounts of urinary extravasation are usually not significant as long as they do not become infected. Since there is no features of infection, we do ureteric stenting. Percutaneous drainage is done only for lacerations.

American association of the Surgery of Trauma (AAST) grading of renal injury

- **Grade I:** Contusion or non-enlarging subcapsular perirenal hematoma, and no laceration
- **Grade II:** Superficial laceration <1 cm depth and does not involve the collecting system (no evidence of urine extravasation), non-expanding perirenal hematoma confined to retroperitoneum
- **Grade III:** Laceration >1 cm without extension into the renal pelvis or collecting system (no evidence of urine extravasation)
- **Grade IV:**
  - Laceration extends to renal pelvis or urinary extravasation
  - Vascular: Injury to main renal artery or vein with contained hemorrhage
  - Segmental infarctions without associated lacerations
  - Expanding subcapsular hematomas compressing the kidney
- **Grade V:**
  - Shattered kidney

- Avulsion of renal hilum: Devascularization of a kidney due to hilar injury
- Ureteropelvic avulsions
- Complete laceration or thrombus of the main renal artery or vein.

Note: Advance one grade for bilateral injuries up to grade III.

12. Management of 4 cm size renal staghorn calculus.

A. Extracorporeal shock wave lithotripsy (ESWL)
B. Percutaneous nephrolithotomy (PCNL)
C. Pyeloplasty
D. Open pyelolithotomy

ANS. **B**

- Management of renal calculi
- Stones <6 mm—conservative treatment
- Stones from 6 mm to 2 cm:ESWL
- Stones >2 cm: PCNL
- For stones at lower renal calyx: Do PCNL
- For staghorn calculi: ESWL+PCNL (Sandwich technique)

Shapes of urinary stones

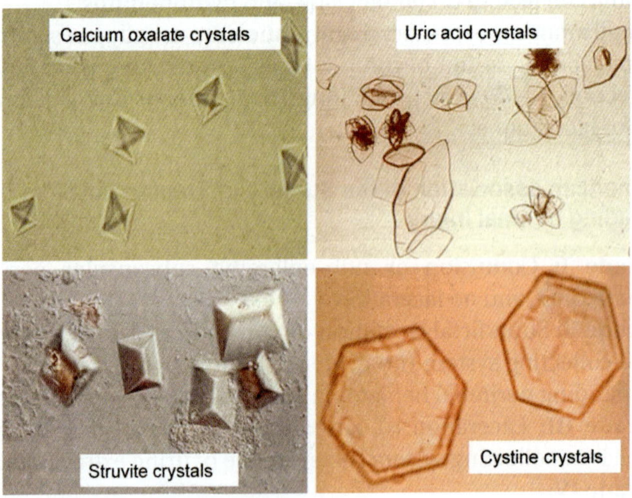

Leucine stones—spherical-shaped
Tyrosine stones—needle-shaped

13. Tumor lysis syndrome is characterized by all, *except*:

A. Hyperuricemia
B. Hypercalcemia
C. Hyperkalemia
D. Hypophosphatemia

ANS. **B**

Cairo-Bishop definition for tumor lysis syndrome

In 2004, Cairo and Bishop defined a classification system for tumor lysis syndrome.

- **Laboratory tumor lysis syndrome**: Abnormality in two or more of the following, occurring within three days before or seven days after chemotherapy.
  - Uric acid > 8 mg/dL or 25% increase
  - Potassium > 6 mEq/L or 25% increase
  - Phosphate > 4.5 mg/dL or 25% increase
  - **Calcium < 7 mg/dL or 25% decrease**
- **Clinical tumor lysis syndrome**: Laboratory tumor lysis syndrome plus one or more of the following:
  - Increased serum creatinine (1.5 times upper limit of normal)
  - Cardiac arrhythmia or sudden death
  - Seizure

A grading scale (0–5) is used depending on the presence of laboratory TLS, serum creatinine, arrhythmias, or seizures.

Howard definition

In 2011, Howard proposed a refinement of the standard Cairo-Bishop definition of TLS accounting for two limitations:

- Two or more electrolyte laboratory abnormalities must be present simultaneously to be considered related to TLS. In fact, some patients may present with one abnormality, but later another one may develop that is unrelated to the TLS (e.g. hypocalcemia associated with sepsis).
- A 25% change from baseline should not be considered a criterion since such increases are rarely clinically important unless the value is already outside the normal range.

Moreover, any symptomatic hypocalcemia should constitute clinical TLS.

14. Nasogastric tube length is measured by:

A. Nose to ear to midpoint between xiphisternum and umbilicus
B. Nose to ear to xiphoid process
C. Nose to umbilicus
D. Nose to ear to pubic symphysis

ANS. **B**

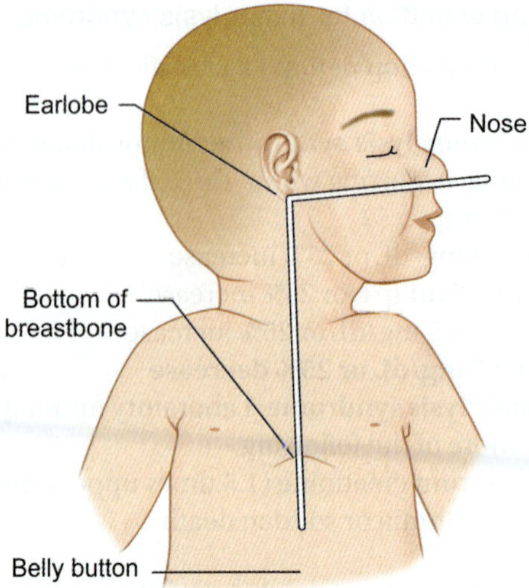

The standard length of the tube in adults are 110 cm and 130 cm.

15. Blister formation in burns is due to involvement of which layer?

A. Epidermis B. Dermis
C. Papillary dermis D. Reticular dermis

ANS. **C**

- First degree burn: Only epidermis is involved
- Second degree burn: Epidermis + part of dermis is involved
  - Superficial second degree—upper part of dermis is involved
  - Deep second degree—extends up to reticular layer
- Third degree burns: involves full dermis
- Fourth degree burns: involves subcutaneous fat and deep structures.

Other important topics in surgery

Instruments

Monopolar cautery (blue-coagulation, yellow-cautery)

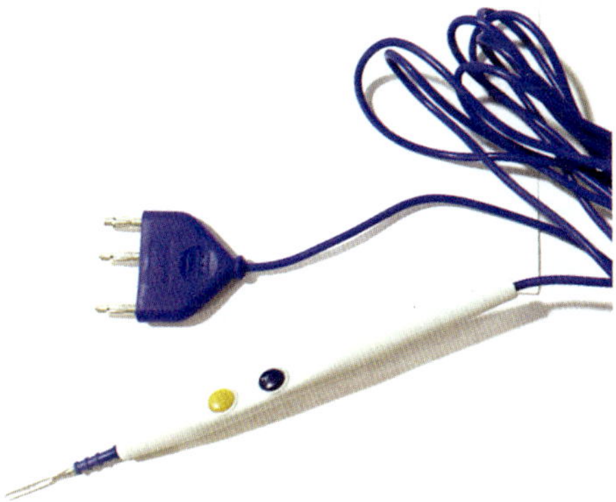

Bipolar cautery

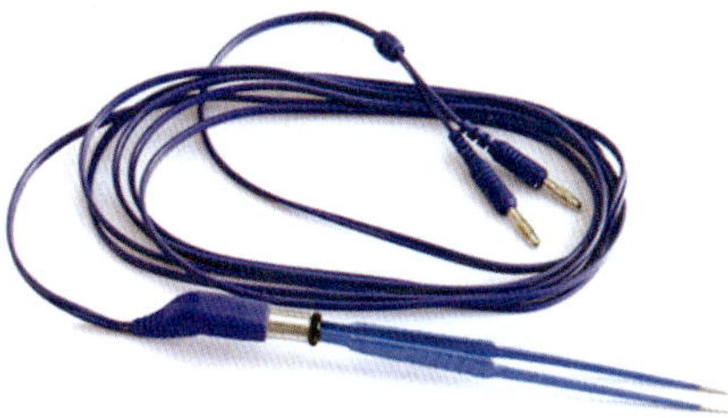

Harmonic scalpel

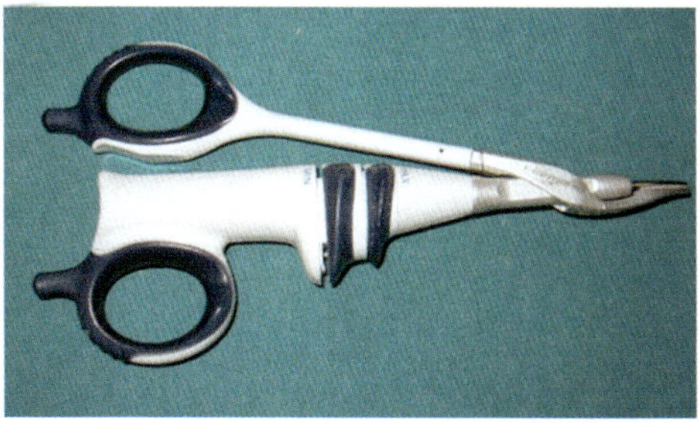

Stapler for hemorrhoidectomy

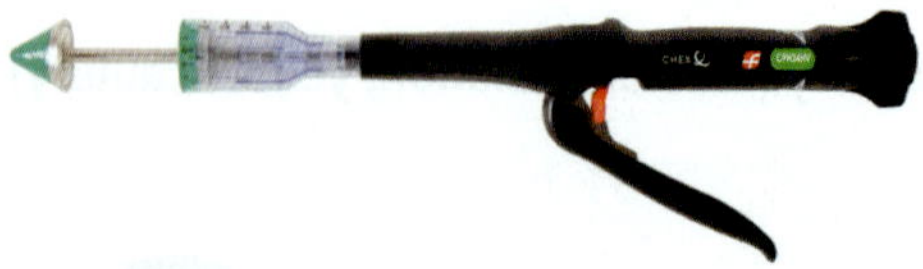

Humby knife for skin grafting

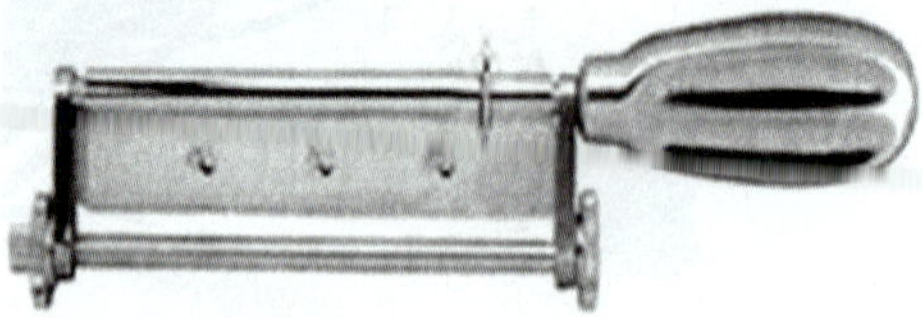

Self-retaining thyroid retractor (Joule's)

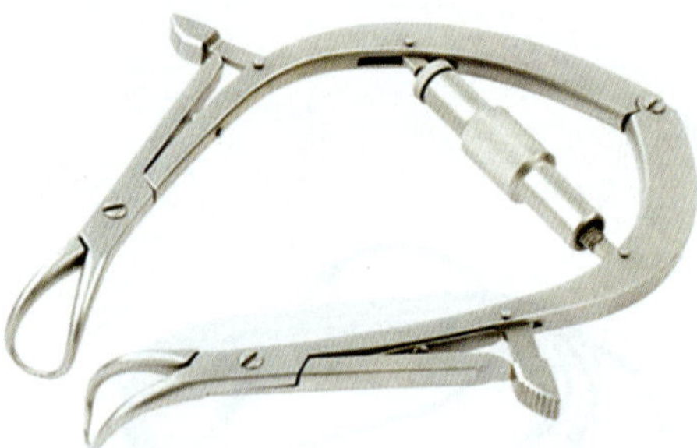

Important surgical positions

Trendelenburg position

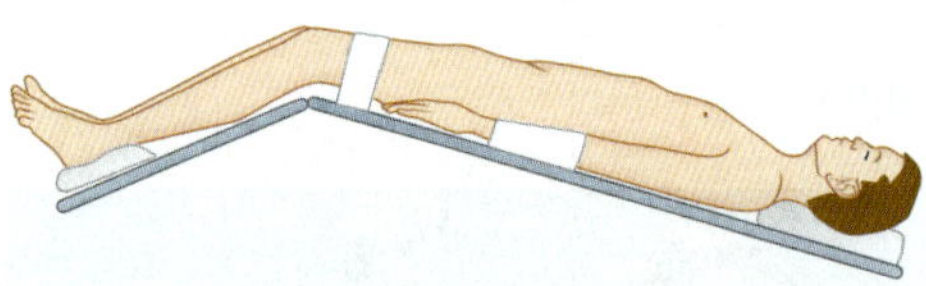

Reverse Trendelenburg position

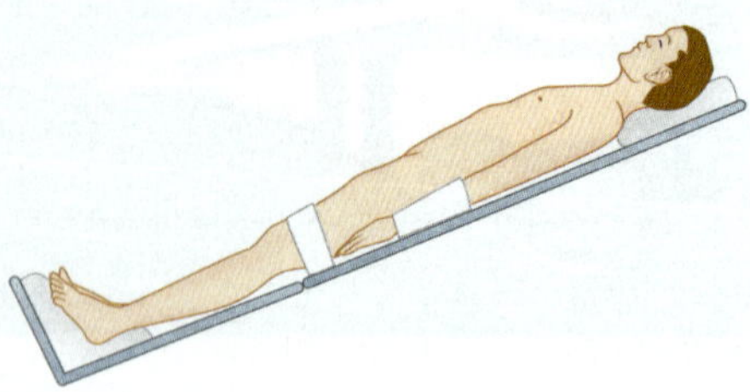

Fowler's position (risk of venous embolism)

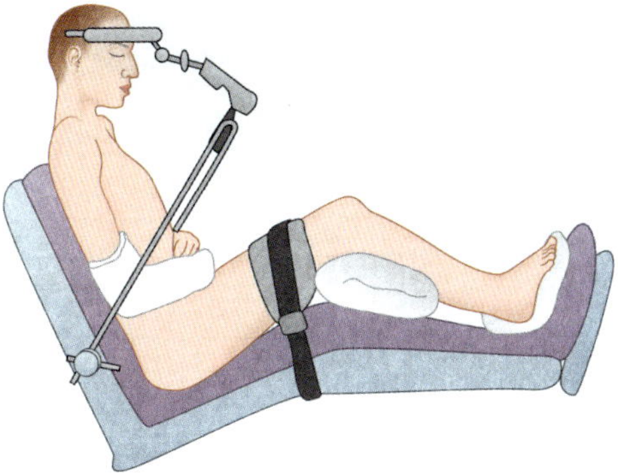

Jack knife position (risk of positional asphyxia)

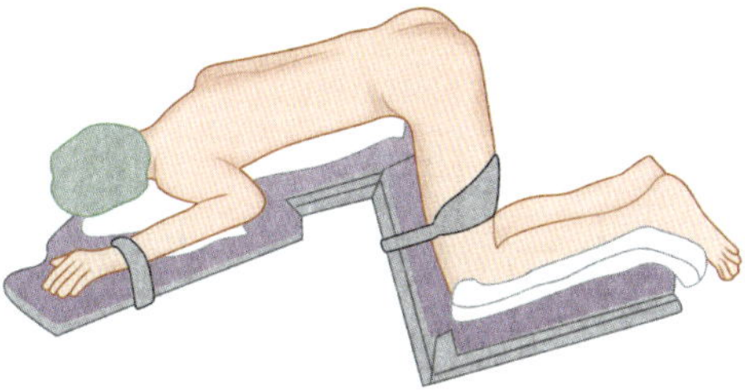

Zones of retroperitoneal hemorrhage

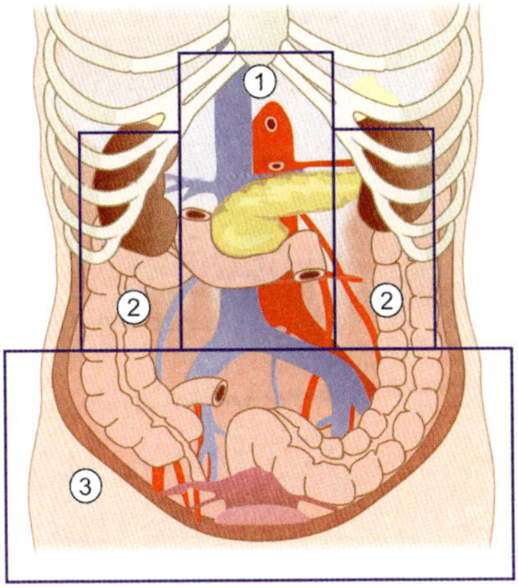

Managementof zone 1 bleed: Explore
Management of zone 2 and 3: Angiography and conservative management

Zones of penetrating neck injury

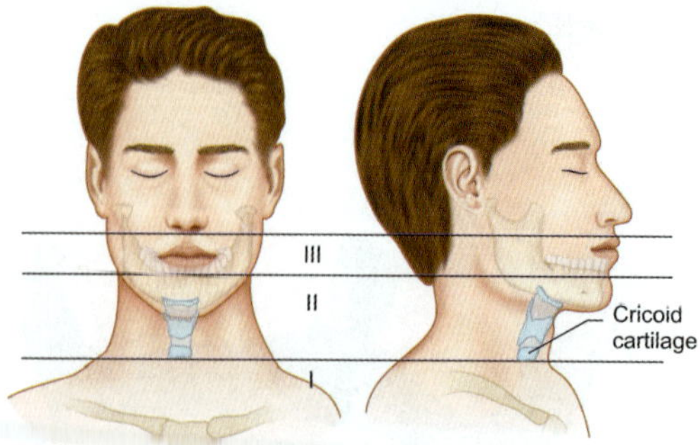

Management of zone 1 and zone 3 injury: Angiography
Management of zone 2 injury: Explore

Sutures

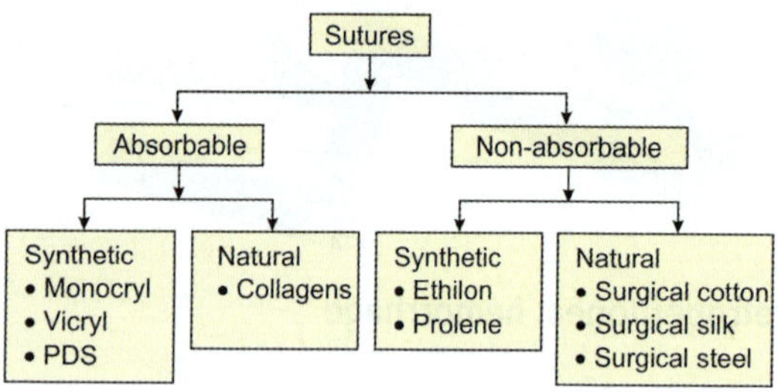

Abbreviation: PDS, polyglyconate

Holding of needle

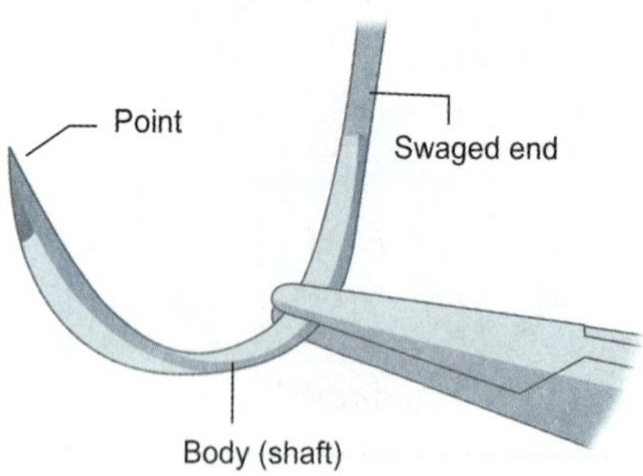

10
CHAPTER

Orthopedics

1. Talocalcaneonavicular joint is a type of:

A. Saddle	B. Ball and socket
C. Hinge	D. Plane

ANS. **B**

Types of joints

1. Synovial joint (freely moveable)
   - Hinge joint : Elbow, ankle, interphalangeal joints
   - Ellipsoid joint : Wrist, all MCPs, atlanto-occipital
   - Pivot : Superior and inferior radioulnar, atlanto-axial
   - Condylar joint : Knee, temporomandibular joint of jaw
   - Saddle point : Thumb (first CMS), sternoclavicular, calcaneocuboidal, incudomalleolar joint
   - Ball and socket : Shoulder, hip, talocalcaneonavicular, incudostapedial joint
   - Arthrodial (plane) joint : Superior (proximal) tibiofibular joint
2. Fibrous joint (immovable)
   - Sutures of skull
   - Syndesmosis: Bones are connected by the interosseous ligament, e.g. distal tibiofibular joint, foot plate of stapes with oval window (tympanostapedial syndesmosis)
   - Gomphosis (peg and socket joint), e.g. tooth in its socket
3. Cartilaginous joint (Partially moveable)
   - **Primary (synchondrosis/hyaline cartilage joint):** Joint between epiphysis and diaphysis of growing/long bones,

spheno-occipital joint, first chondrosternal, costochondral joints.

- **Secondary (symphysis of fibrocartilaginous joint):** Symphysis pubis, manubriosternal joint, intervertebral joints, and sacrococcygeal joints.

2. The following injury shows:

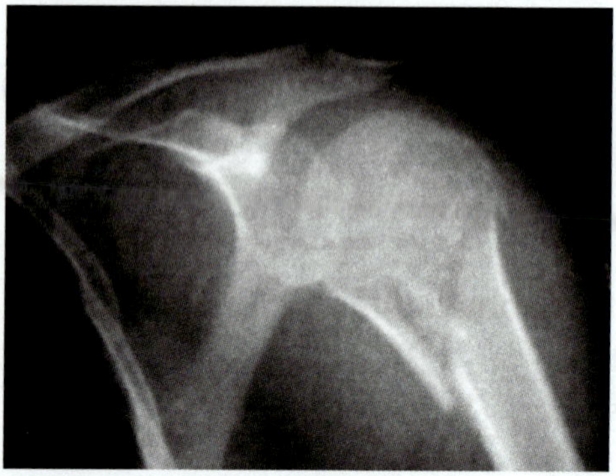

A. Gardner's classification type 2
B. Neer's classification type 3
C. Gartland classification type 4
D. Masons type 3

ANS. **B**

Classification	*Fracture*
Allman	Clavicle
Rockwood	Acromioclavicular injury
Neer	Proximal humerus
Gartland	Supracondylar fracture
Mason	Head of radius
Frykman, Fernandez, Melone	Distal end of radius
Tiles	Pelvis fracture
Judet	Acetabular fracture
Pipkins	Head of femur
Anatomical, Pauwel, Gardener	Neck of femur
Hawkins	Neck of talus
Essex-Lopresti	Calcaneum

3. All of the followings are true about Sprengel's deformity, *except:*

A. Associated with congental scoliosis
B. Associated with diastematomyelia
C. High incidence with Klippel-Feil syndrome
D. Associated with dextrocardia

ANS. **D**

Sprengel's deformity: It is congenital elevation of the scapula.

Is a complex deformity of the shoulder and the most common congenital shoulder anomaly.

Associations of Sprengel's deformity:

- Klippel-Feil syndrome
- Spina bifida
- Diastematomyelia
- Torticollis
- Kyphoscoliosis

Klippel-Feil syndrome

The most common sign of the disorder is restricted mobility of the neck and upper spine. A short neck and low hairline at the back of the head may occur in some patients.

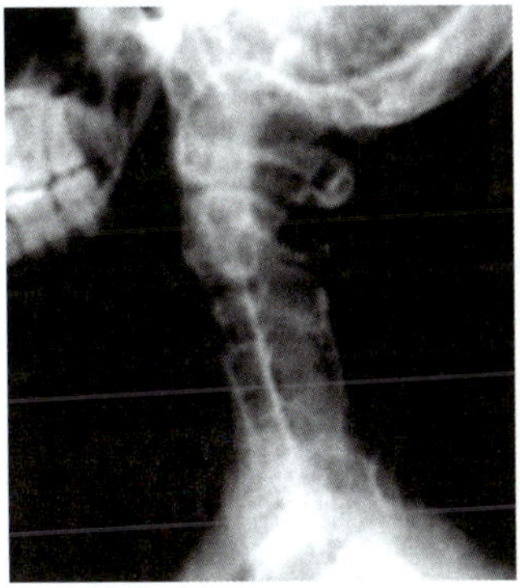

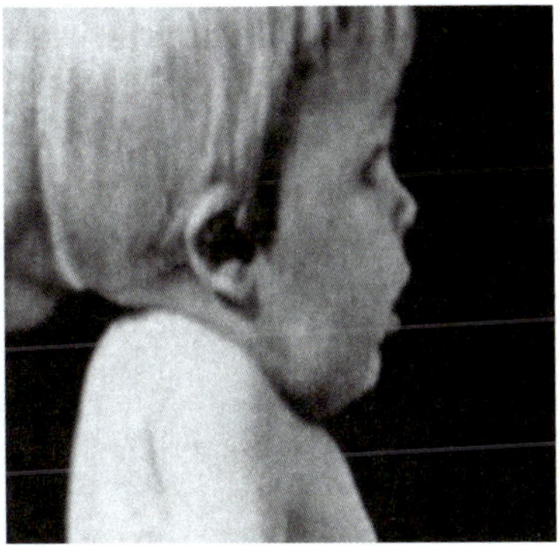

4. A patient with history of RTA is seen at emergency department. He has an open injury of Gustilo-Anderson type III B. What does this indicate?

A. Bilateral limb wound >10 cm with extensive laceration
B. Bilateral limb wound of size <1 cm
C. Bilateral limb wound >10 cm with extensive soft tissue damaged periosteal strip

D. Wound between 1 and 10 cm in length, without extensive soft tissue damage, flaps or avulsion

ANS. **C**

Gustilo and Anderson classification system of open fractures	
Classification	*Description*
Type 1	• Puncture wound of less than or equal to 1 cm with minimal soft tissue injury • Minimal wound contamination or muscle crushing
Type 2	• Wound is greater than 1 cm in length • Moderate soft-tissue injury • Soft tissue coverage of the bone is adequate • Comminution is minimal
Type 3a	• Extensive soft tissue damage • Includes massively contaminated, serverely • comminuted, or segmental fractures • Soft tissue coverage of the bone is adequate
Type 3b	• Extensive soft tissue damage with periosteal stripping and bone exposure • Usually severely contaminated and comminuted • Flap coverage is required to provide soft tissue coverage
Type 3c	• Associated with an arterial injury requiring repair for limb salvage

5. A patient came with complains of lower limb weakness. Examiner places one hand under the patient's heel and patient is then asked to raise his other leg against downward resistance. What is the test being performed?

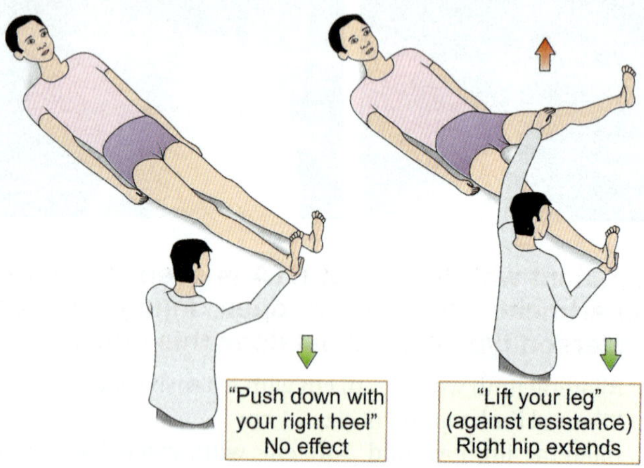

A. Hoover's test
B. McBride test
C. Waddell's test
D. Lachman test

ANS. **A**

Hoover's test: Patient is asked to perform a unilateral straight leg raise.

Positive test is inability to lift the leg due to neuromuscular weakness. Another finding is examinor does not feel increased pressure in the palm that underlies the raising leg.

6. X-ray shows:

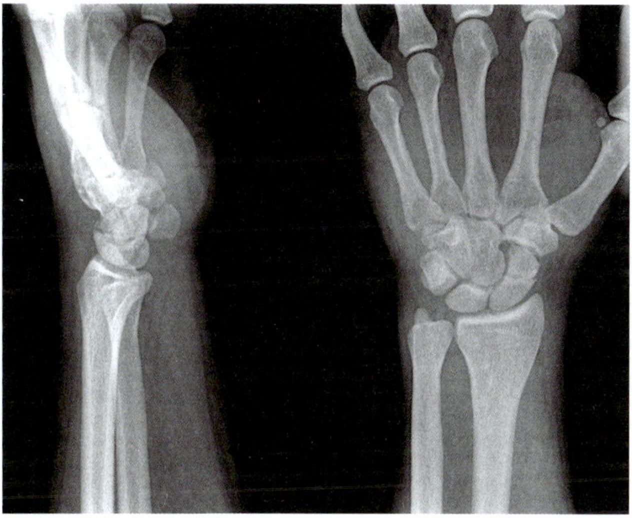

A. Fracture scaphoid
B. Fracture scaphoid and perilunate dislocation
C. Perilunate dislocation
D. Colles fracture

ANS. **A**

This is an isolated fracture scaphoid. The main differential was the option of scaphoid and perilunate dislocation.

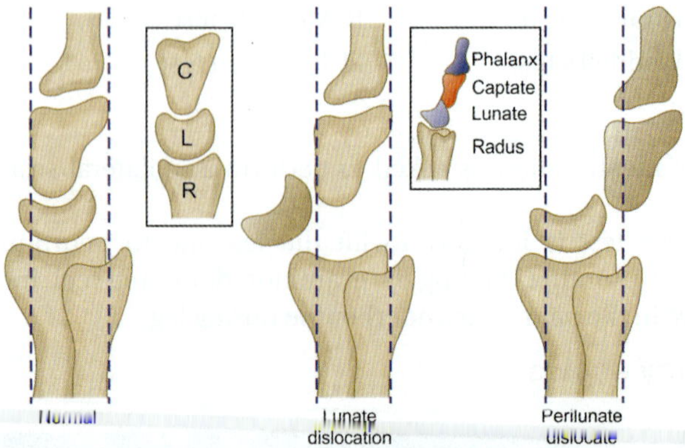

In the X-ray provided, the alignment of radius, lunate and capitate is maintained. Hence, the answer is isolated fracture scaphoid.

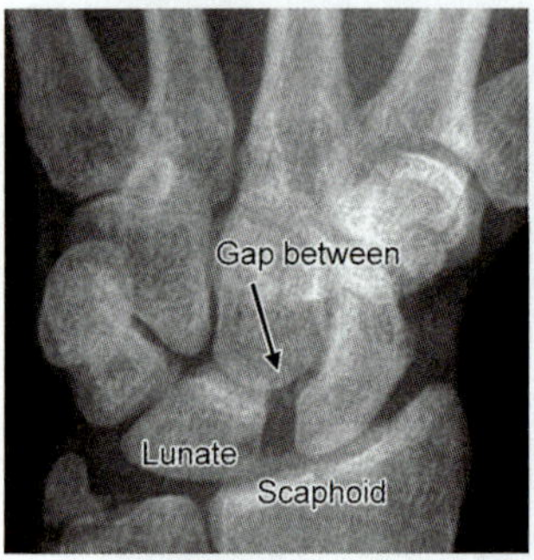

This abnormal gap in the lunate and scaphoid is seen on X-ray has been compared to famous smiles with similarly impressive gaps

British comedian Terry Thomas

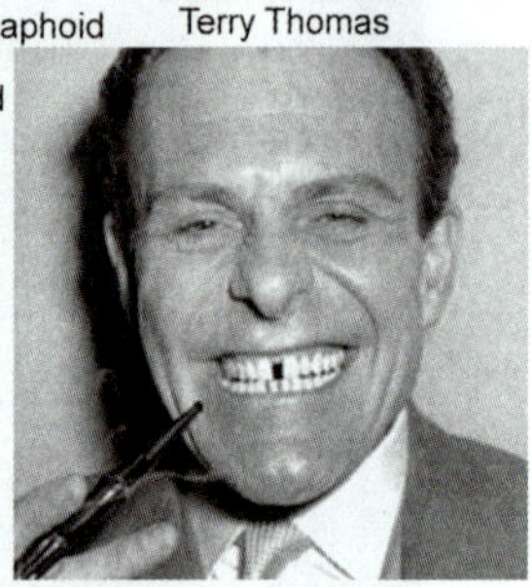

Important tables to revise for AIIMS

1. Test for muscles around shoulder joint

Test	*Muscle tested*
Lift off test	Subscapularis
Jobe test	Supraspinatus
Speed test	Biceps
Yergason test	Biceps
Belly press test	Subscapularis

2. Test for nerve injury

Signs of nerve injury	
Froment's sign	Ulnar nerve injury
Egawa test	Ulnar nerve injury
Card test	Ulnar nerve injury

Contd...

Contd...

Ape thumb deformity	Median nerve injury
Wrist drop	Radial nerve injury
Pointing index sign	Median nerve injury
Claw hand	Combined ulnar and median nerve injury

3. Splints used in orthopedics

Splint	*Indication*
Aeroplane splint	Axillary nerve injury
Knuckle Bender splint	Ulnar nerve injury
Cock-up splint	Radial nerve injury
Functional humeral brace	Humerus shaft fractures
Volkmann's splint/turn buckle splint	Volksmann's ischemic contracture (VIC)

4. Tractions in orthopedics

Smith and Dunlop	Supracondylar fracture
Bryant, Russell, Gallows, Fisk, 90-90	Fracture shaft of femur
Agnes Hunt	Fixed flexion deformity hip
Well Leg traction	Abduction/adduction deformity hip
Milwaukee, Boston, Lyon	Scoliosis
SOMI Brace (Sternal Occipital Mandibular Immubilizer)	For cervical spine
Minerva	C spine
Von Rosen splint	Developmental dysplasia of hip
Dennis Brown	Congenital talipes equinovarus

5. Avascular necrosis of bones

Name	*Bone*
Kienbock's disease	Lunate
Perthes disease	Femoral head
Panner's disease	Capitulum
Preiser's disease	Scaphoid
Johansson-Larsen disease	Osteochondritis of lower pole of patella
Freiberg disease	Osteochondritis of 5th metatarsal head
Scheuermann's disease	Ring apophysis of vertebra
Kohler disease	Navicular
Sever's disease	Calcaneal tuberosity
Osgood-Schlatter disease	Tibial tubercle

11

CHAPTER

Social and Preventive Medicine

1. Child-Pugh score is a type of:

A. Nominal B. Ordinal
C. Quantitative D. Continuous

ANS. **B**

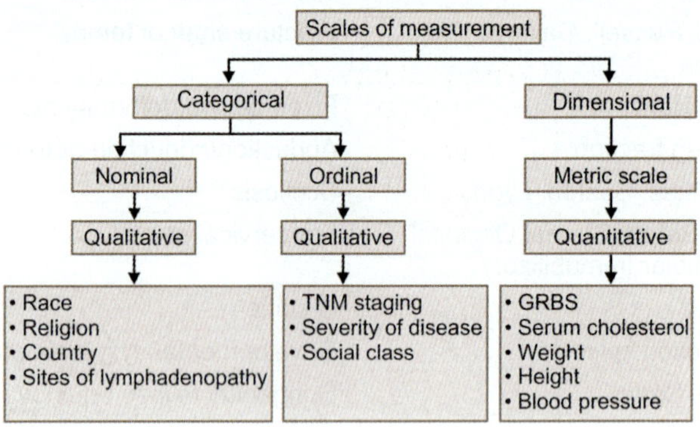

Child-Pugh score

Clinical and laboratory criteria	*Points*		
	1	*2*	*3*
Encephalopathy	None	Mild to moderate (grade 1 or 2)	Severe (grade 3 or 4)
Ascites	None	Mild to moderate (diuretic responsive)	Severe (diuretic refractory)
Bilirubin (mg/dL)	<2	2–3	>3
Albumin (g/dL)	>3	2.8–3.5	<2.8

Contd...

Contd...

Prothrombin time			
• Seconds prolonged	<4	4–6	>6
• International normalized ratio	<1.7	1.7–2.3	>2.3
Child-Turcotte-Pugh class obtained by adding score for each parameter (total points) • Class A = 5 to 6 points (least severe liver disease) • Class B = 7 to 9 points (moderately severe liver disease) • Class C = 10 to 15 points (most severe liver disease)			

2. An unvaccinated child came at 18 months of age to your clinic, what vaccination should be taken?

A. BCG, OPV and DPT
B. Pentavalent only
C. BCG, OPV
D. DPT booster and OPV

ANS. **D.**

If the child is unvaccinated, principles to be followed for the vaccines given in options are:
- Maximum age up to which BCG can be given is 1 year
- Maximum age up to which pentavalent can be given is 1 year
- Maximum age up to which DPT can be given is 7 years
- Maximum age up to which OPV can be given is 5 year.

3. Crude birth rate (CBR) of a village is 20, how many pregnancies are registered in that subcenter?

A. 100
B. 120
C. 80
D. 60

ANS. **D**

- Population of a subcenter is 5,000.
- So, for a CBR of 20, number of births = (20/1000) × 5000 = 100.

There is a pregnancy wastage (abortion) of 10%, so corrected total no. of pregnancies = 100 + 10 = 110

But, at a given amount of time, only 50% pregnancies are registered. So, the final answer is 55.

4. Mid-day meal has:

A. 1/2 of protein and 1/3 of energy
B. 1/3 of energy and 1/2 of protein
C. 1/2 of protein and 1/2 of energy
D. 1/4 of energy and 3/4 of carbohydrate.

ANS. **A**

This is a direct question.

Mid-Day Meal Program

- **Supplements**—1/3 of total energy and 1/2 of total protein requirements.
- Also called school health program
- Launched in 1961
- It is under ministry of health.

5. In a statistical study for calculating the effect of drug on patient's sugar level, the test showed significant difference when in reality there was no difference:

A. Alpha error
B. Beta error
C. Gamma error
D. Power of a test

ANS. **A**

Type 1 error (alpha error):
- Indicates false positivity
- Drug actually does not work, but we think that it works
- So, we reject the null hypothesis even if it is correct.

Type 2 error (beta error):
- Drug really works, but we think that it would not
- So we accept the null hypothesis even if it is incorrect.

Power of a test = 1 - beta error

6. Prevalence rate of leprosy in India is:

A. 0.66/10000
B. 9.3/10000
C. 0.66/100000
D. 9.3/100000

ANS. **A**

A total of 86,000 **cases** were on record as on April 1, 2014, giving a **prevalence rate** (PR) of 0.68 per 10,000 population.

India alone accounted for 58.85% of the global **leprosy** burden.

World Leprosy day—**World Leprosy Day** is observed internationally on January 30 or its nearest Sunday to increase the public awareness of the Leprosy or Hansen's Disease.

Annual case detection rate of leprosy is 9.71/1 lakh.

7. Which are the following are correctly matched:

1. Red—moribund
2. Green—needs ICU care
3. Yellow—needs observation
4. Black—OP consultation

A. 1
B. 2
C. 3
D. 4

ANS. **C**

Color codings in triage:

- *Red (immediate):* Are used to label those who cannot survive without immediate treatment but who has a chance of survival.
- *Yellow (observation):* For those who require observation. Their condition is stable for the moment, they are not in immediate danger of death.
- *Green (wait):* Reserved for walking wounded, who will require medical care at some point, after more critical injuries have been treated.
- *Black (expectant):* Are used for the deceased and for those whose injuries are so extensive that they will not be able to survive given the care that is available.

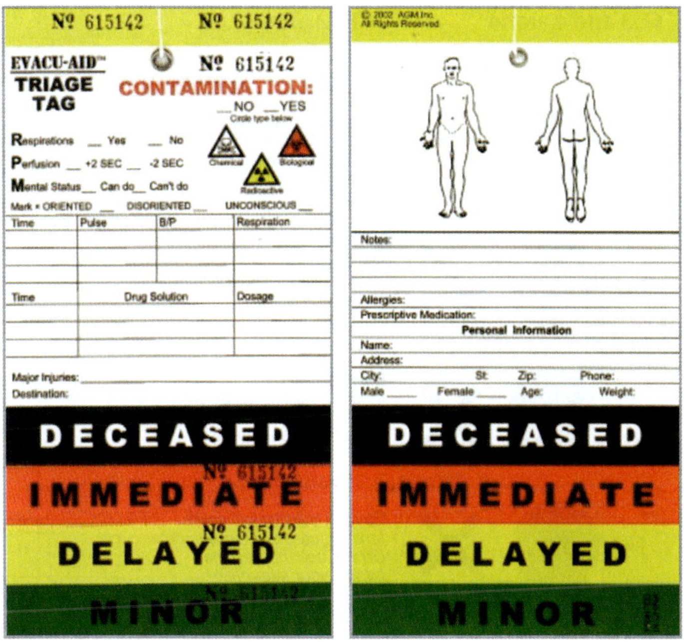

8. Which of the following vaccines can be used:

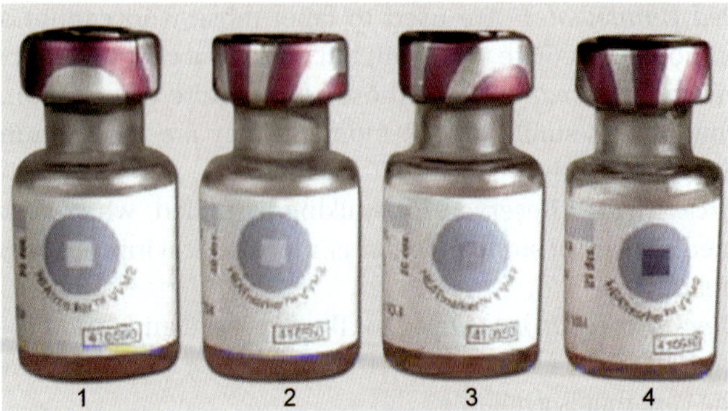

A. 1 and 2 alone   B. 1 alone
C. 3 and 4 alone   D. 2 alone

ANS. **A**

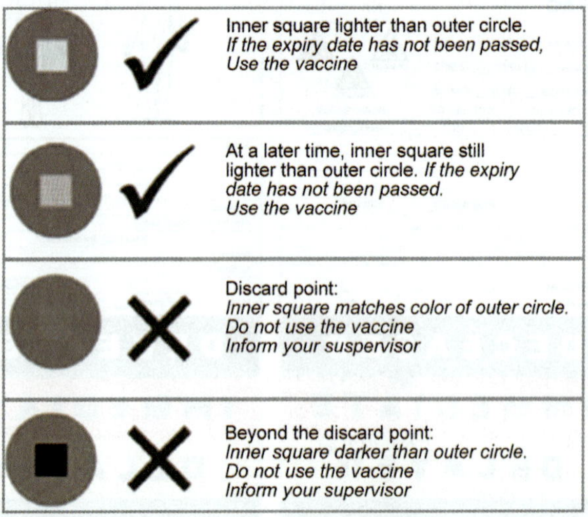

9. High sensitivity in a study means:

A. If the disease is rare, then it means that patient is definitely having it.
B. High chance of having a disease if the prevalence is high
C. High chance of definitely having the disease
D. High chance of not getting the disease.

ANS. **B**

Truth

Test result	Disease (number)	Non-disease (number)	Total (number)
Positive (number)	***A*** (True negative)	***B*** (False negative)	$T_{\text{(Test positive)}}$
Negative (number)	***C*** (False negative)	***D*** (True negative)	$T_{\text{(Test negative)}}$
	$T_{\text{(Disease)}}$	$T_{\text{(Non-disease)}}$	Total

- **Sensitivity: A/(A+C) × 100**
  Sensitivity is the probability that a test will indicate 'disease' among those with the disease.
- **Specificity: D/(D+B) × 100**
  Specificity is the fraction of those without disease who will have a negative test result.
- **Positive Predictive Value: A/(A+B) × 100**
  Positive predictive value—diagnostic power of a screening test to correctly identify the disease.
- **Negative Predictive Value: D/(D+C) × 100**
  Negative predictive value—diagnostic power of a screening test to exclude the disease.

Important formulas in SPM

1. Extra edge in sensitivity, specificity
   In sequential testing (one diagnostic test is done, if that test is positive, same test is repeated again):
   - False positivity decreases
   - Specificity increases
   - Sensitivity decreases

   In parallel testing (two different diagnostic tests are done together):
   - False negativity decreases
   - Sensitivity increases
   - Specificity decreases

   (This question was asked in May and November session JIPMER 2017)

2. Normal distribution curve

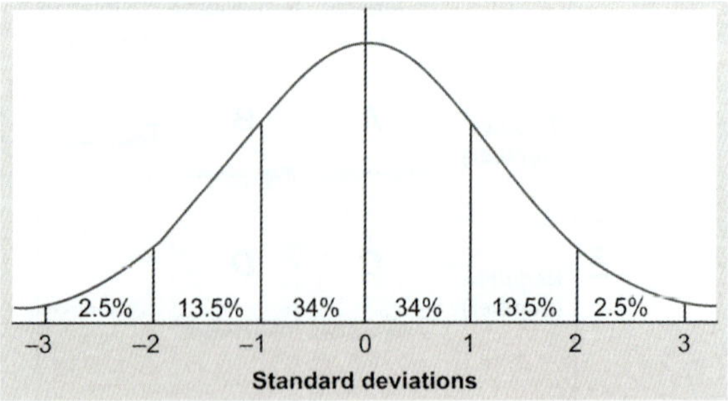

3. Positive and negative skew

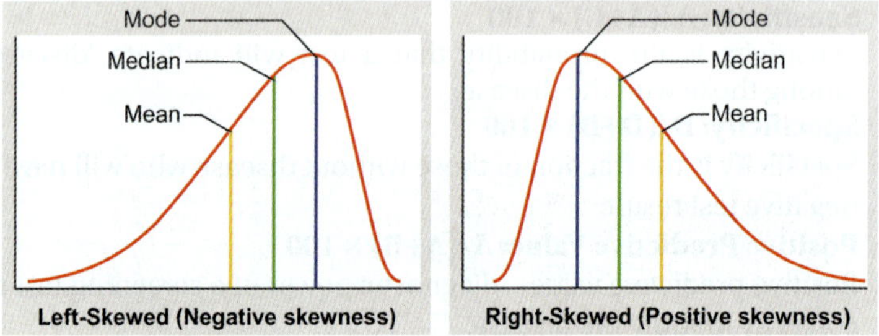

- In positive skew: Mean > Median > Mode
- In negative skew: Mean < Median < Mode

4. Odds ratio = P/(1–P) {where, P is the probablity}.
5. Sample size of a study = $4PQ/D^2$ { where, P = prevalence, Q = (1–P), D is error
6. Standard error of a population=√ (PQ/sample size)
7. Crude birth rate = (8 × total fertility rate) + 1.

12
CHAPTER

Ophthalmology

1. The given image depicts which of the following condition?

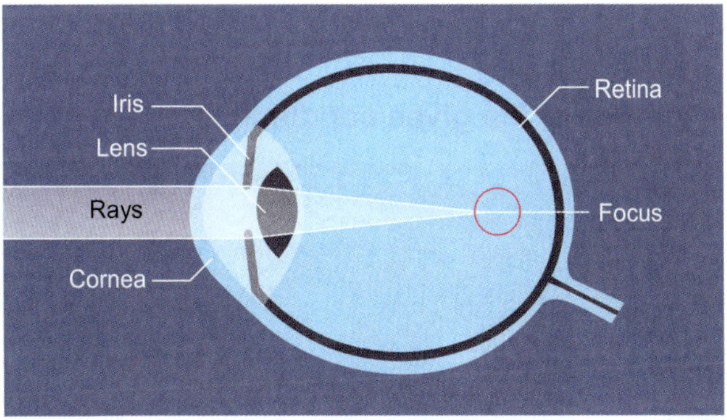

A. Presbyopia B. Hypermetropia
C. Astigmatism D. Myopia

ANS. **D**

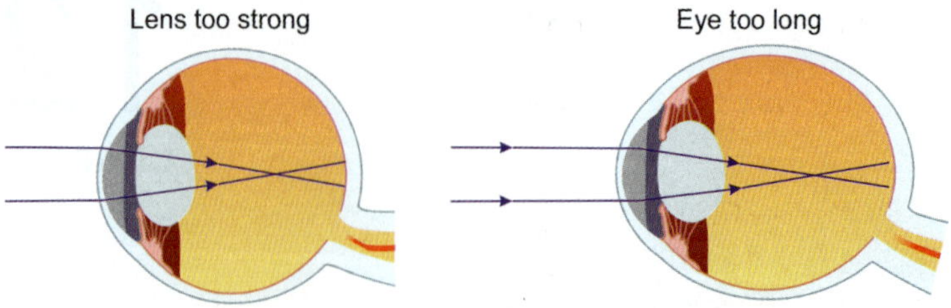

(a) Myopia

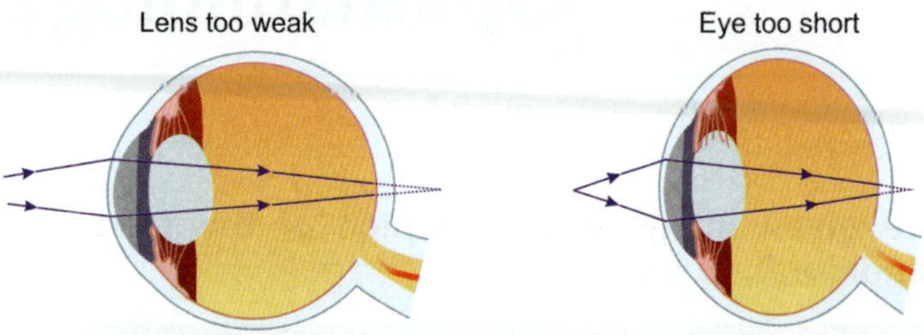

(b) Hyperopia

2. Diagnosis of the given condition is:

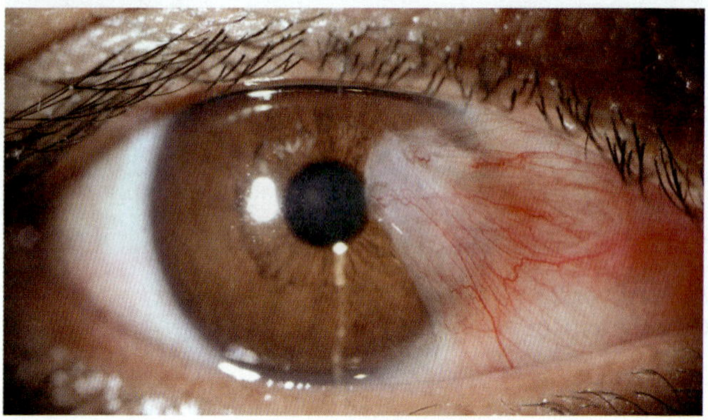

A. Episcleritis
B. Bitot spots
C. Pterygium
D. Pinguecula

ANS. **C**

Given image is that of pterygium.

Pinguecula Bitot's spots episceritis

Pinguecula Bitot's spots Episcleritis

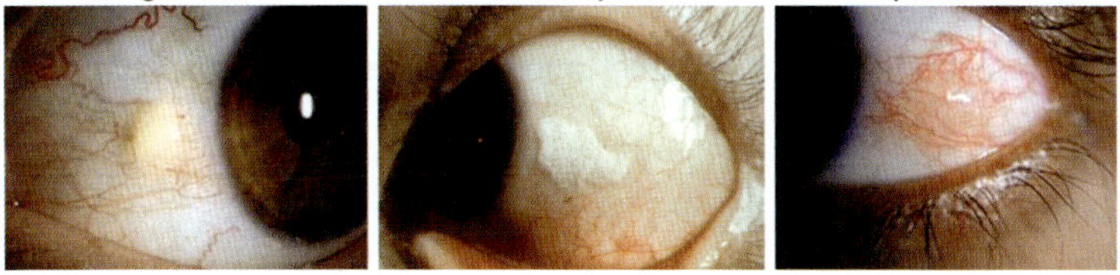

- Pinguecula: Degenerative condition of conjunctiva characterized by triangular yellowish white patch on the bulbar conjunctiva near limbus.
- Pterygium: Growth of conjunctiva—wing-shaped fold of conjunctiva encroaching onto cornea, Stocker's line.

3. Which of the following is not done in endophthalmitis:

A. Topical antibiotics B. Intravenous antibiotics
C. Pars plana vitrectomy D. Intravitreal antibiotics

ANS. **B**

Treatment of endophthalmitis:

1. Pars plana vitectomy
2. Intravitreal antibiotics
3. Topical antibiotics
   Intravenous antibiotics may not be needed for endophthalmitis.

4. The diagnosis of the FFA image shown below is:

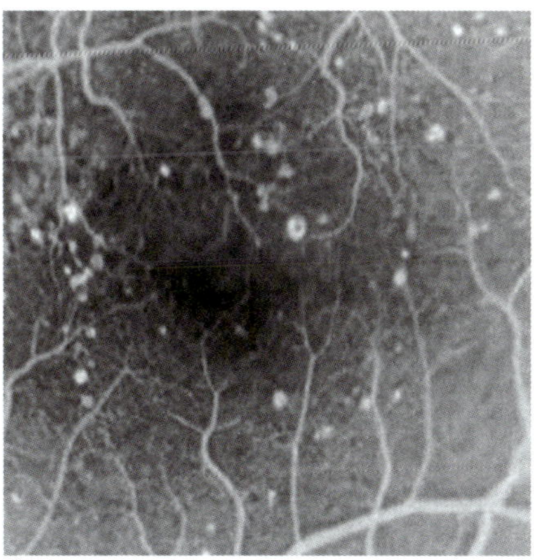

A. Nonproliferative diabetic retinopathy
B. Birdshot choroidopathy
C. Central serous retinopathy
D. Salmon patch

ANS. **A**

The image shows the classical microaneurysm in diabetic retinopathy.

Diabetic retinopathy

- *Most important factor in DR*: Duration of diabetes
- *Second most important factor*: Glycemic factor
- *First fundus examination in DR*: After 5 years
- *Frequency of follow up*: 1 yearly (mild NPDR), 6 monthly (moderate NPDR), 3 monthly (severe NPDR), 2 monthly (PDR).

5. An elderly male who has a history of glaucoma, on examination shows bulging of cornea. What is the diagnosis?

A. Keratoconus
B. Staphyloma
C. Glaucomatous iridocyclitis
D. Keratomalacia

ANS. **B**

Staphyloma is an abnormal protrusion of the uveal tissue through a weak point in the eyeball. There are 5 types of staphyloma.

1. Anterior staphyloma
2. Intercalary
3. Ciliary
4. Equatorial
5. Posterior.

6. Most common lacrimal gland tumor is:

A. Non-Hodgkin's lymphoma
B. Pleomorphic adenoma
C. Adenoid cystic tumor
D. Squamous cell carcinoma

ANS. **A**

This was a confusing question, because:

- Most common benign lacrimal gland tumor is pleomorphic adenoma
- Most common malignant lacrimal gland tumor is adenoid cystic tumor

- Most common overall tumor is nonepithelial malignancy (non-Hodgkin's lymphoma).

Other important images in ophthalmology

Schiotz (indentation) tonometry

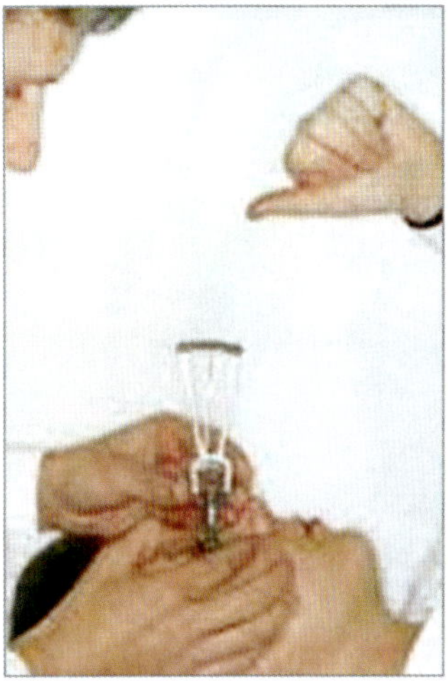

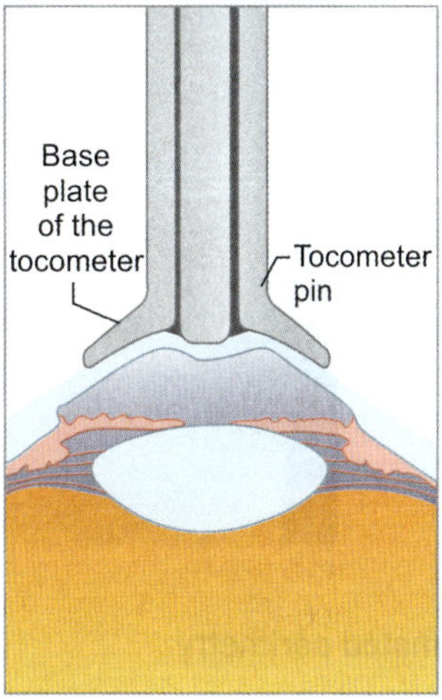

Applanation tonometry

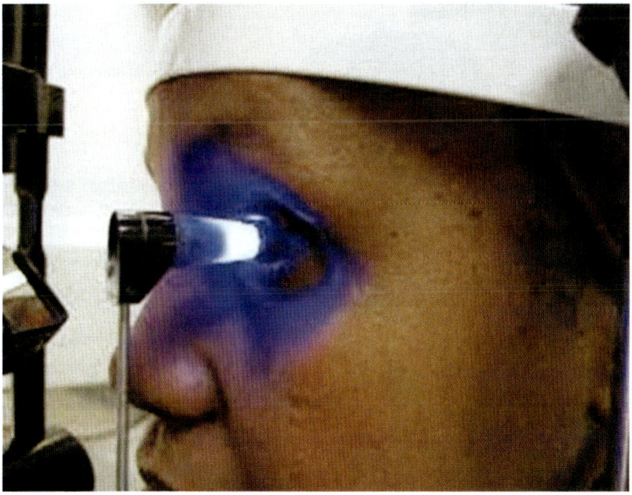

Self (rebound) tonometry

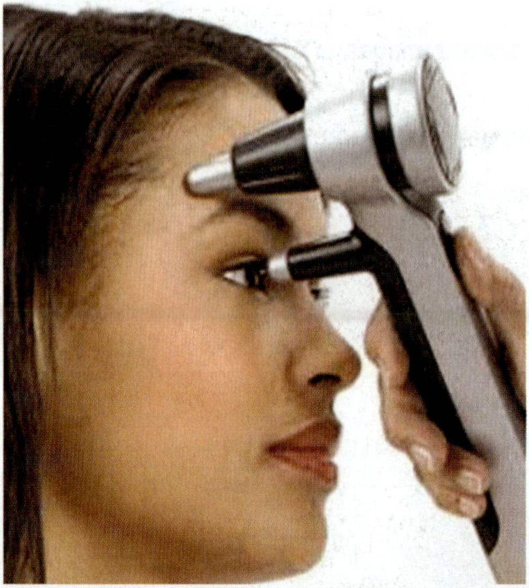

Automated perimetry

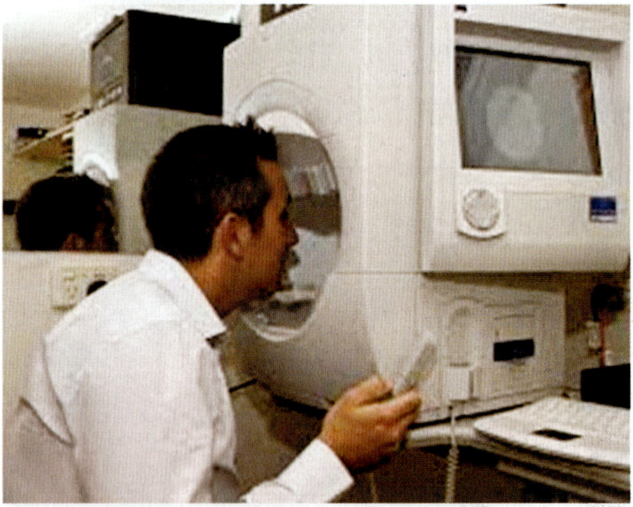

A scan

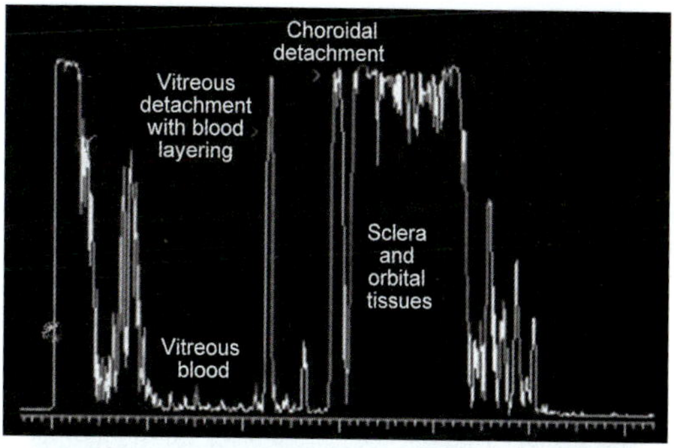

B scan

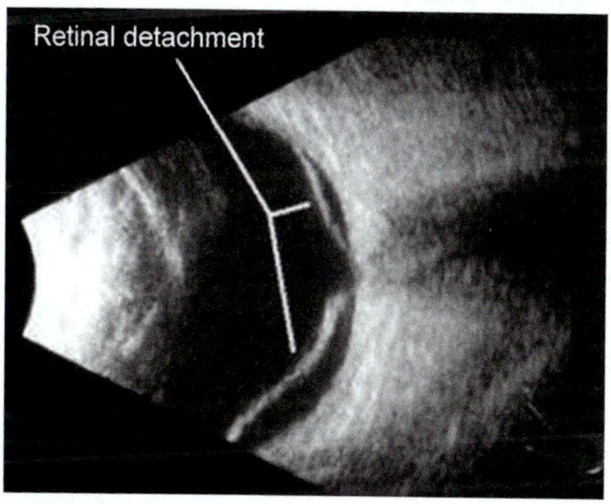

Structure of intraocular lens

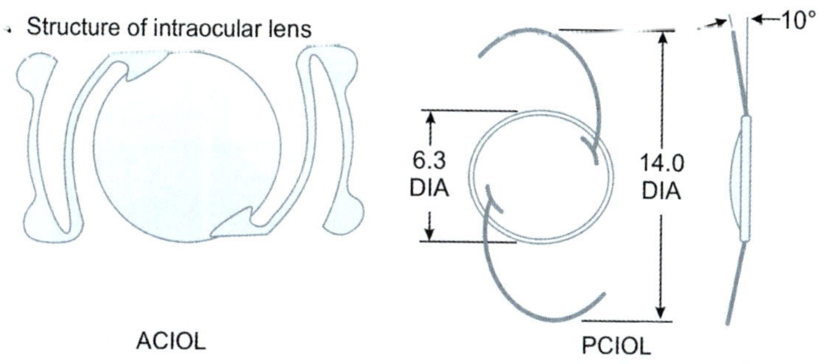

Abbreviations: ACIOL, anterior chamber intraocular lens; PCIOL, posterior chamber intraocular lens.

Iris claw lens

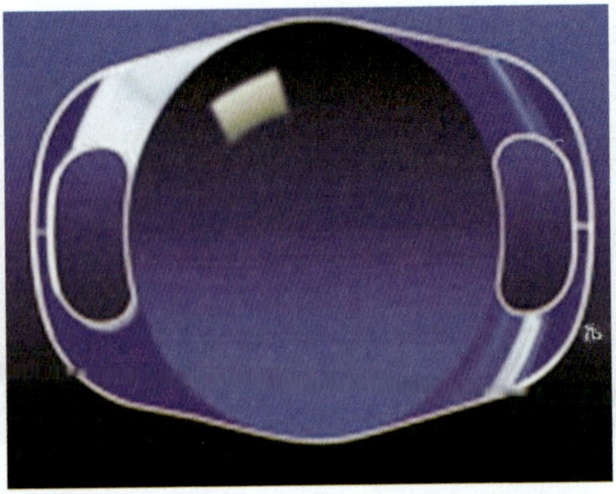

Express glaucoma implant

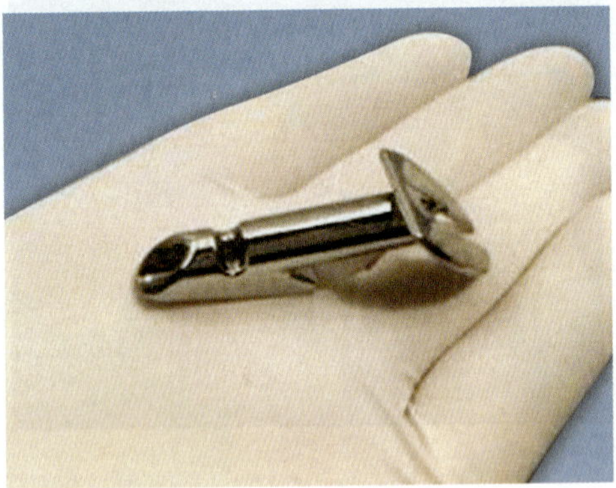

AGV implant for glaucoma

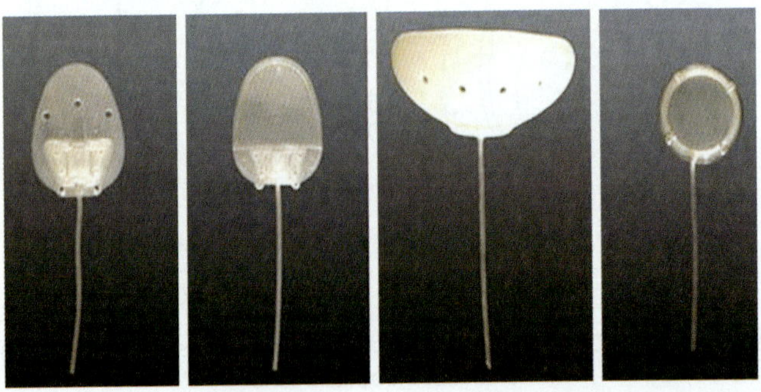

Keratometry

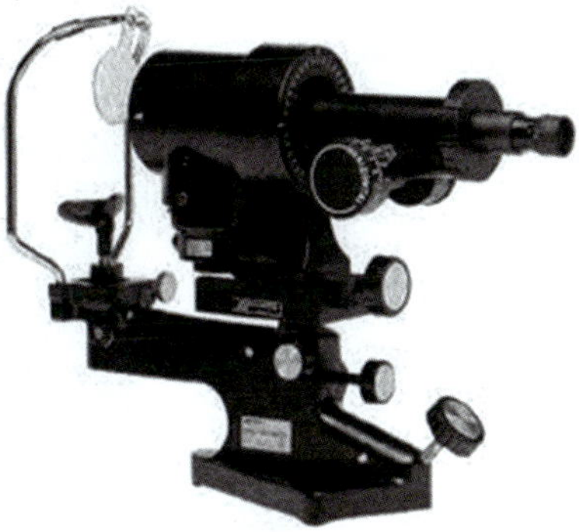

Specular microscopy

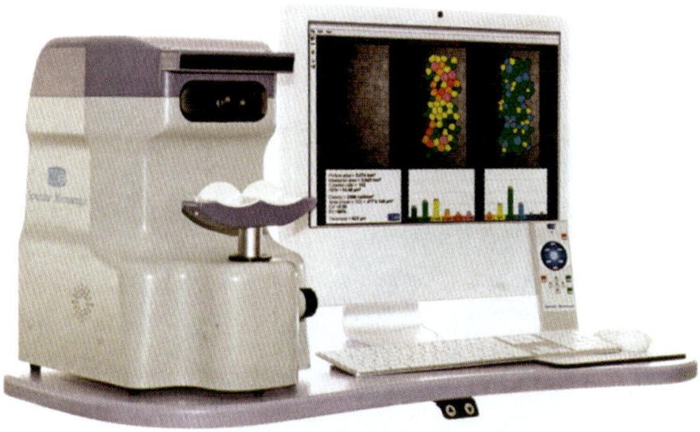

Corneal esthesiometry

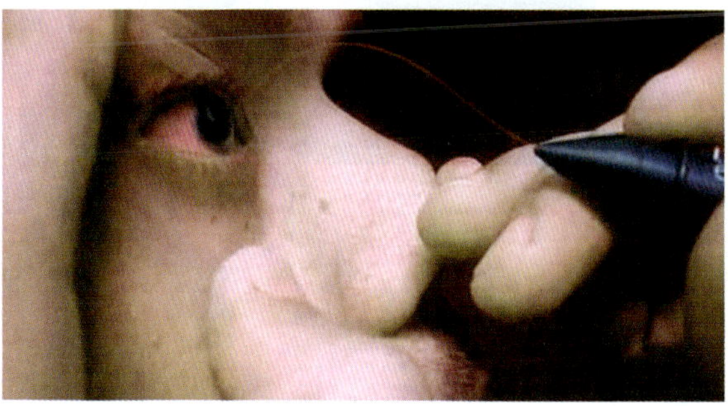

Corneal pachymetry

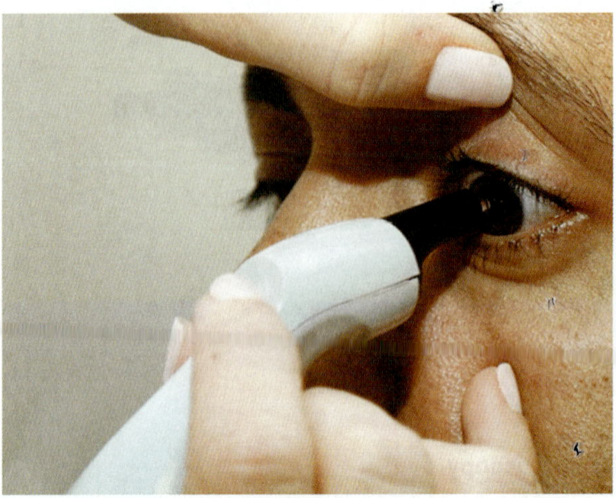

Indirect ophthalmoscopy

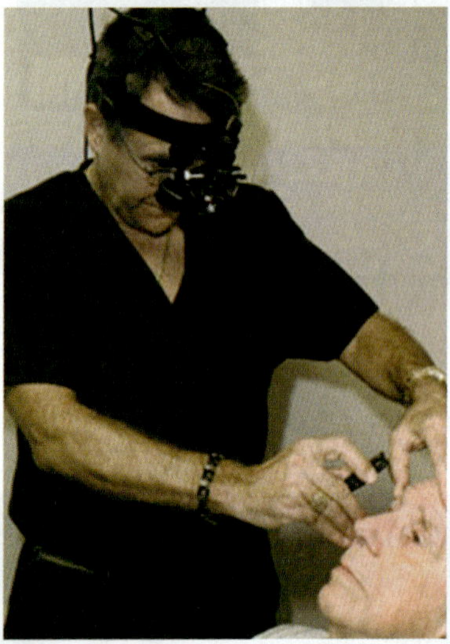

Direct ophthalmoscopy

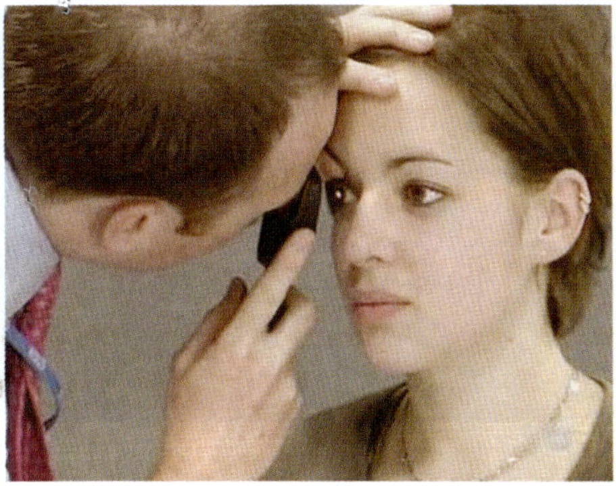

Slit lamp microscopy

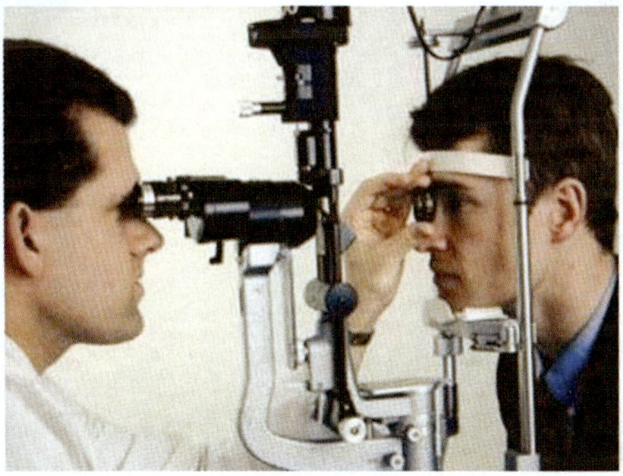

Synoptophore for squint

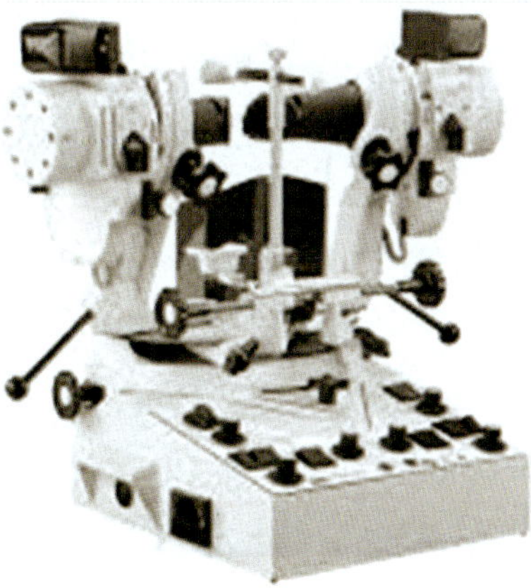

Optical coherence tomography (OCT)

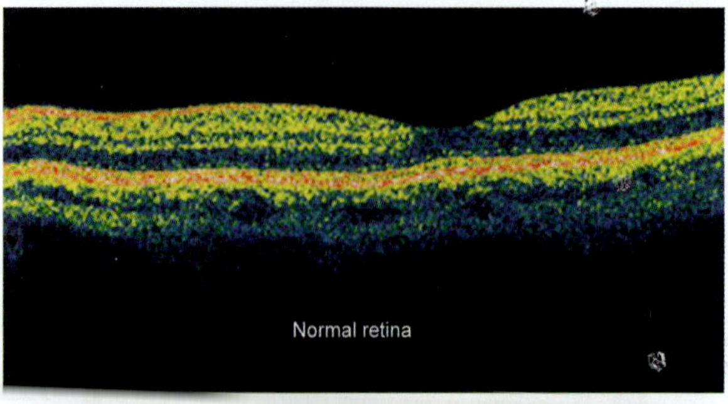

FFA image of CSR (ink-blot pattern)

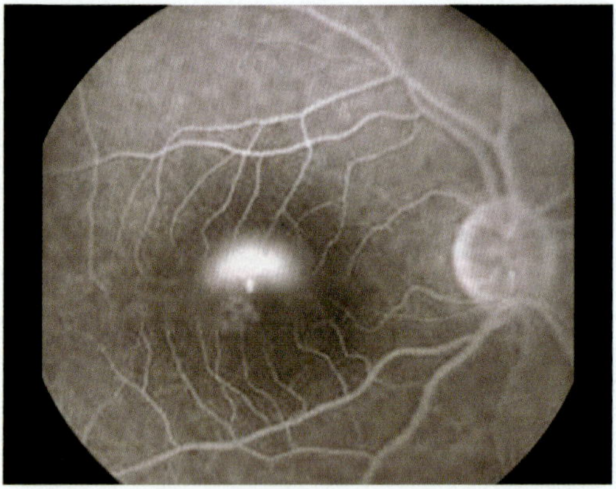

FFA image of honeycomb pattern

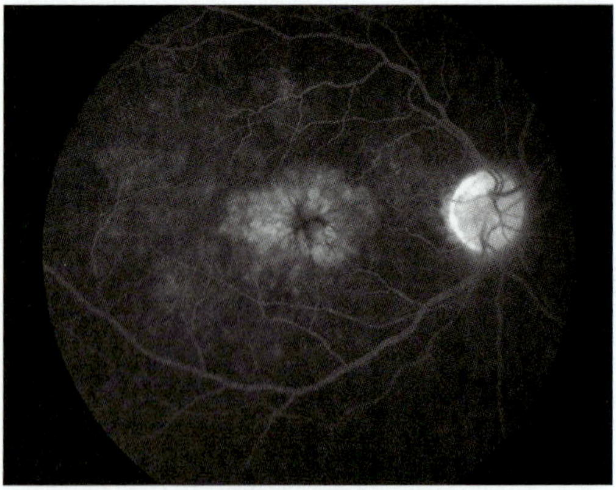

Christmas tree pattern in myotonic dystrophy

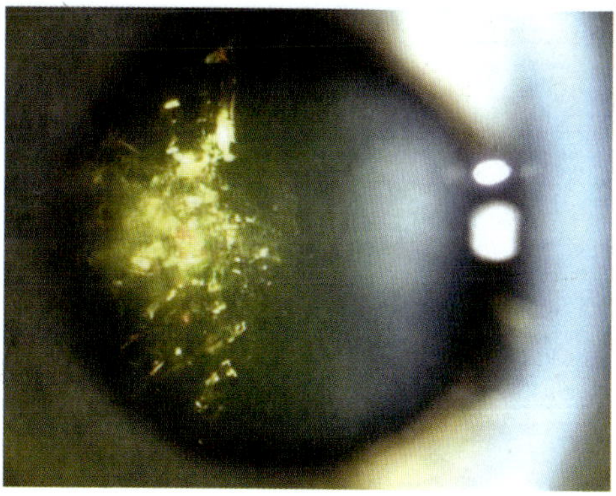

Brushfield's spots in Down's syndrome

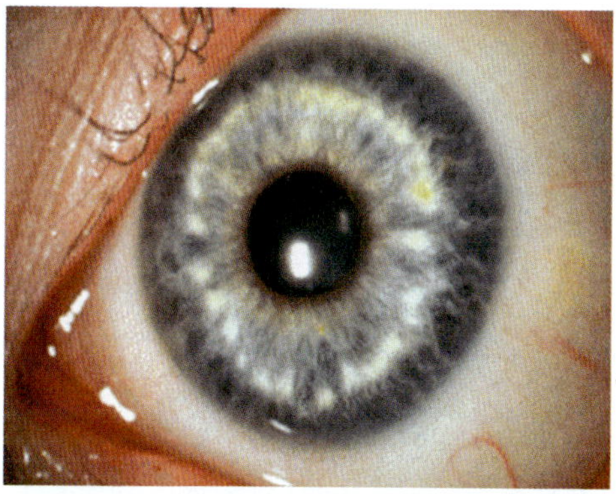

Vortex keratopathy

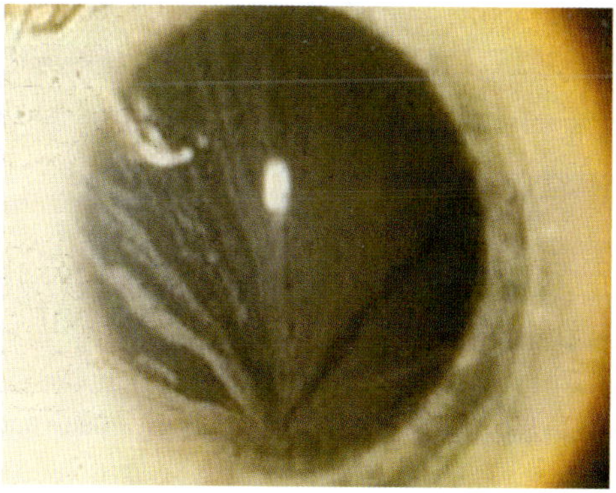

Sunflower cataract

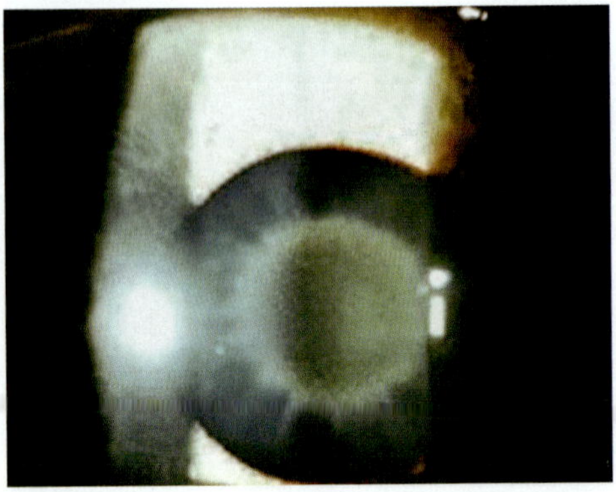

Retinitis pigmentosa

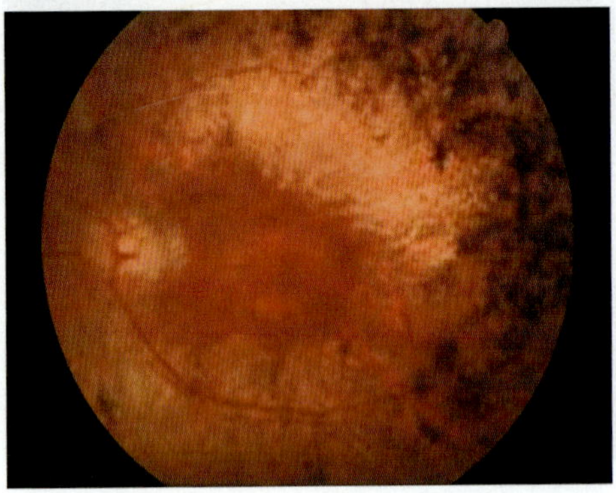

Cherry red spot cattle tracking

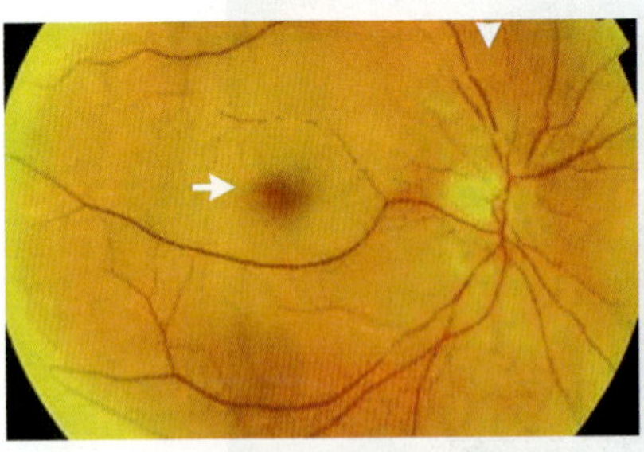

Cherry red spot

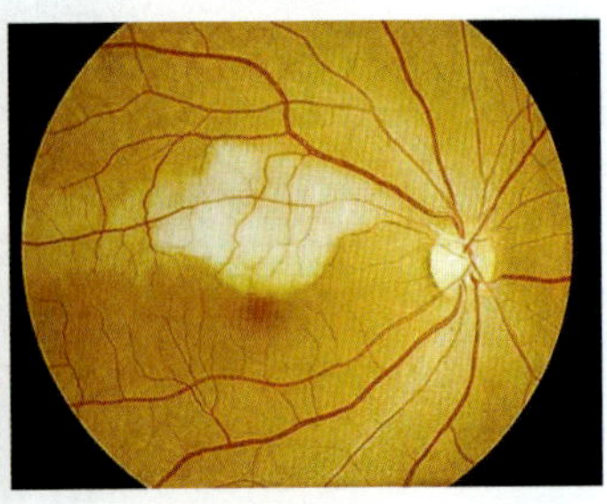

Cattle tracking

Roth spots

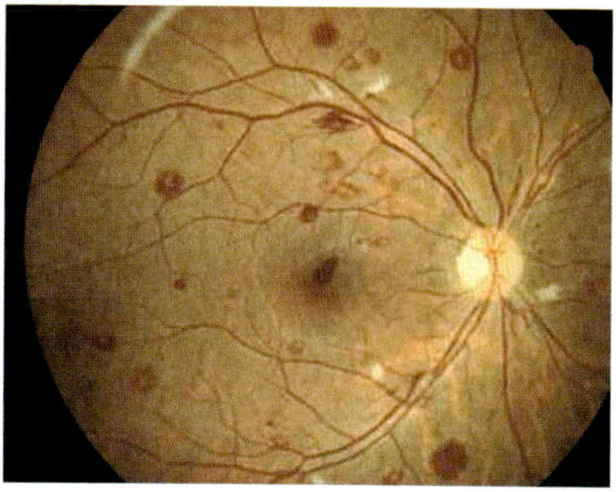

CMV retinitis (pizza pie and cottage cheese pattern)

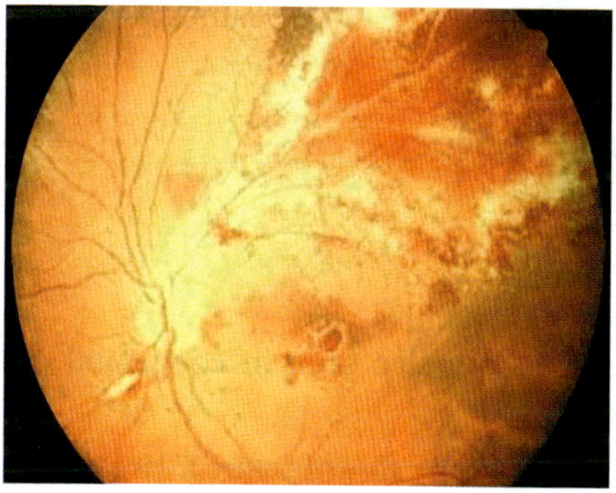

Lisch nodule

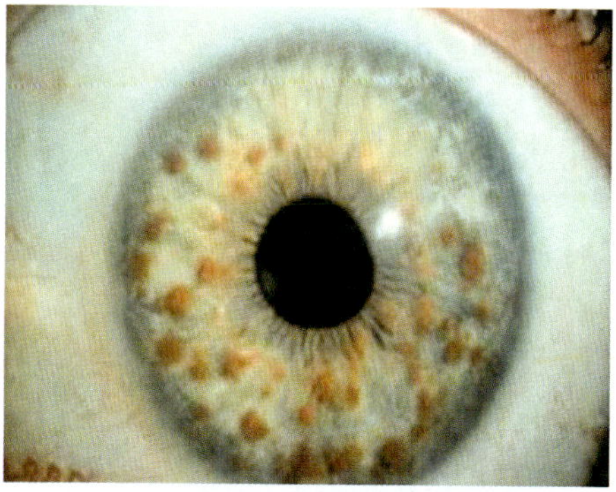

13
CHAPTER

Dermatology

1. Hutchinson's triad include all *except:*

A. Hutchinson's teeth B. Mulberry molar
C. Interstitial keratitis D. Deafness

ANS. **B**

Hutchinson triad include:
1. Hutchinson teeth
2. Mulberry molar
3. Interstitial keratitis

- Seen in congenital syphilis.
- Mulberry molars are also seen in congenital syphilis, but not included in triad.

2. A 35-year-old man developed a brown pigmentation on the face after taking nonsteroidal anti-inflammatory drug (NSAID) for fever, joint pain and malaise. What is the diagnosis?

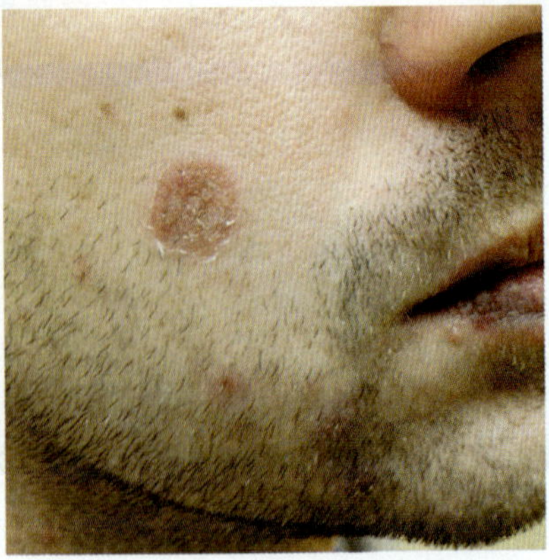

A. Dengue fever B. Chikungunya
C. Fixed drug eruption D. Melasma

ANS. **C**

- The image shows a hyperpigmented lesion, and with the history of drug intake, the diagnosis is fixed drug eruption.

Close differentials of hyperpigmented lesions in face

Malar rash in SLE

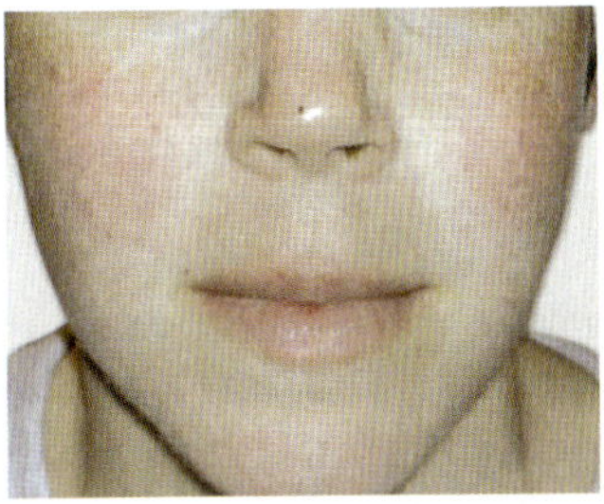

Acne rosacea (note telangiectasia)

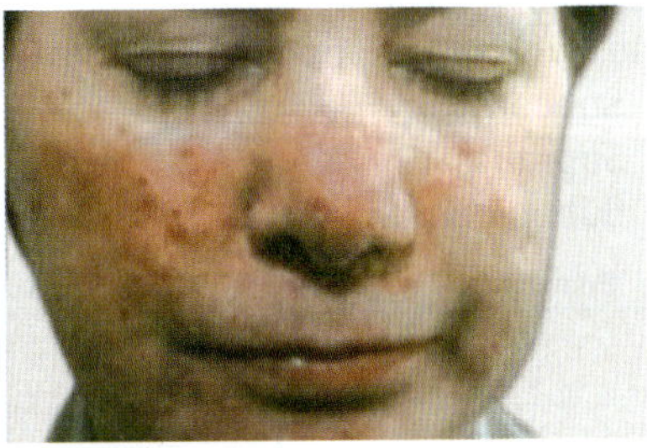

Melasma (brown pigmentation in face)

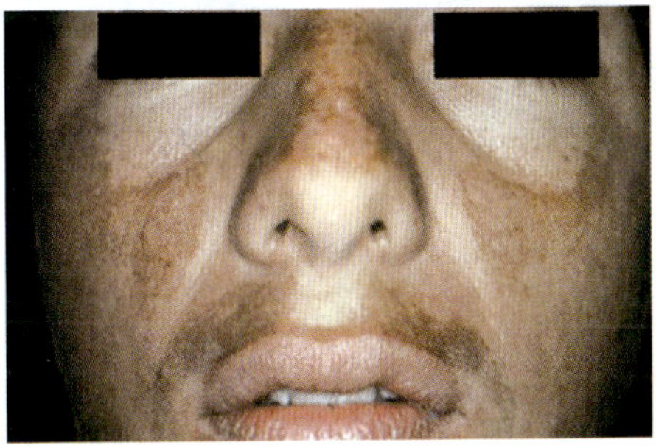

3. Highest concentration of desmosomes are seen in which location?

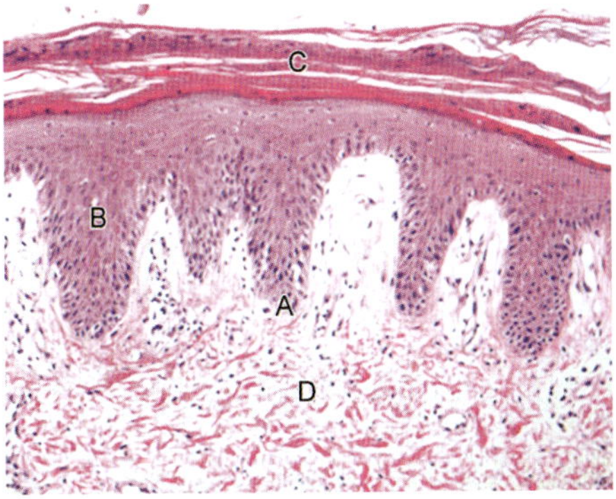

A. A
B. B
C. C
D. D

ANS. **B**

- Desmosomes are maximally seen at suprabasal portion which is marked by B.
- A shows dermoepidermal junction which has abundant hemidesmosomes.

Bullous disorders

The levels of bullous disorders can be:

1. Subcorneal
2. Suprabasal
3. Subepidermal

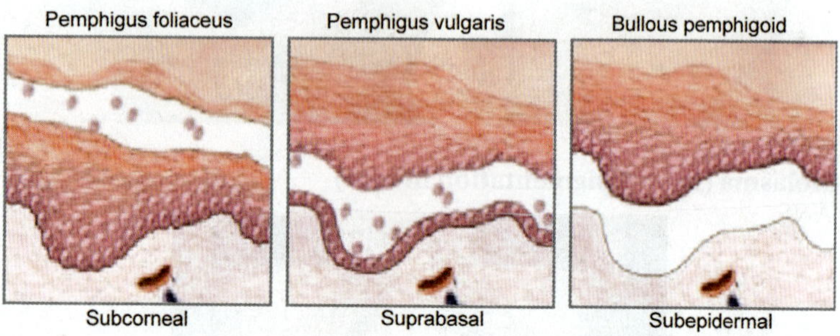

14
CHAPTER

Ear, Nose and Throat

1. Target sign is seen in:

A. Traumatic epistaxis
B. Traumatic cerebrospinal fluid (CSF) rhinorrhea
C. Spontaneous CSF rhinorrhea
D. Petrositis

ANS. **B**

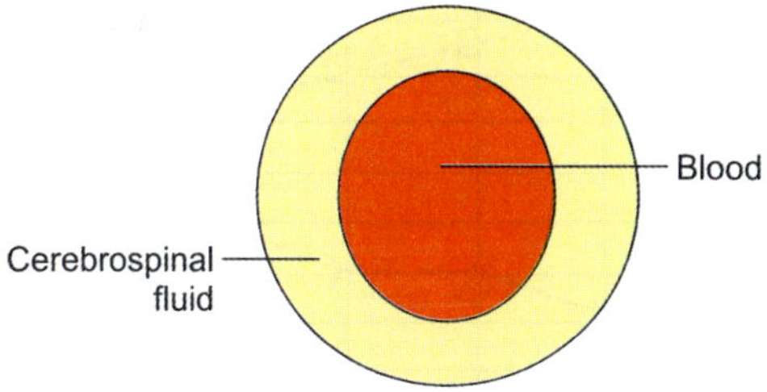

2. A factory worker with history of long standing deafness was evaluated and a diagnosis of noise-induced hearing loss (NIHL) was made. NIHL affects which part of the ear?

A. Macula
B. Semicircular canal
C. Inner hair cells
D. Saccule

ANS. **C**

- Noise-induced hearing loss damages hair cells, starting in the basal turn of cochlea.
- Outer hair cells are affected before the inner hair cells

- Tympanometry classically shows dip at 4000 Hz (Acoustic dip/ Boiler's dip).

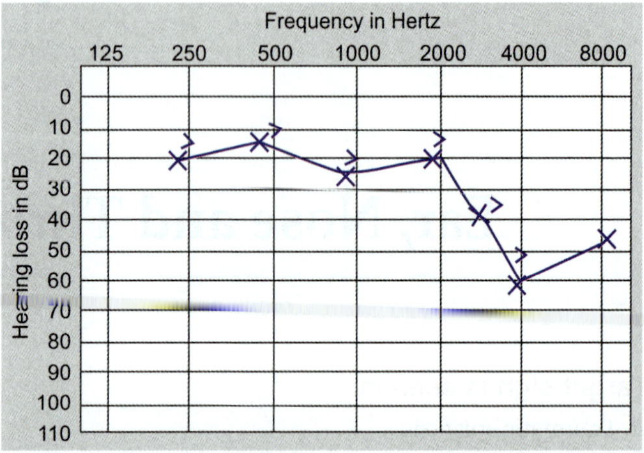

Otosclerosis (Carhart's notch)

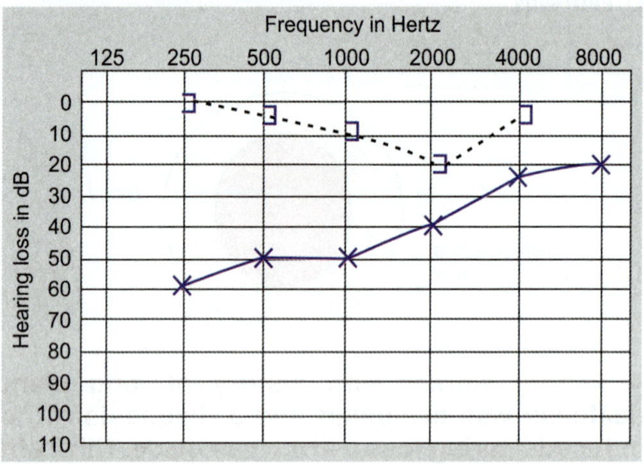

3. Most common causes of recurrent laryngeal nerve palsy is:

A. Bronchogenic carcinoma B. Thyroid surgery
C. Mediastinal tumors D. Pancoast tumor

ANS. **B**

Causes of recurrent laryngeal palsy:

1. Thyroid surgery
2. Neck trauma

3. Carcinoma cervical esophagus
4. Cervical lymphadenopathy
5. Carcinoma apex of lung
6. Carcinoma thyroid

- Most commonly injured is left recurrent laryngeal nerve because of its long course.
- Left recurrent laryngeal nerve winds around arch of aorta and right winds around subclavian trunk to supply all the muscles of larynx except cricothyroid sensory supply of larynx below the vocal cord.

Important Images in ENT

Cochlear implant

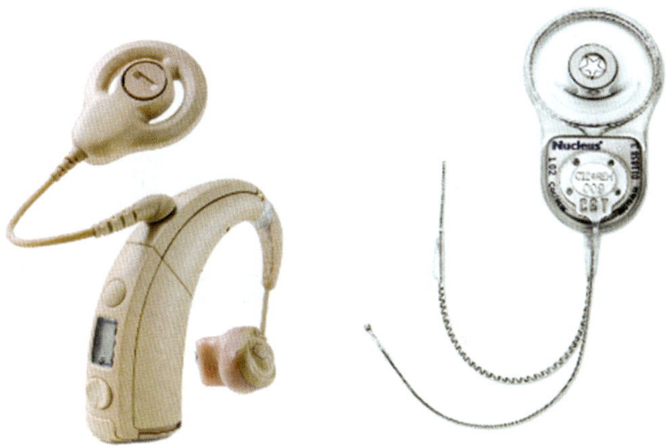

Auditory brainstem implant

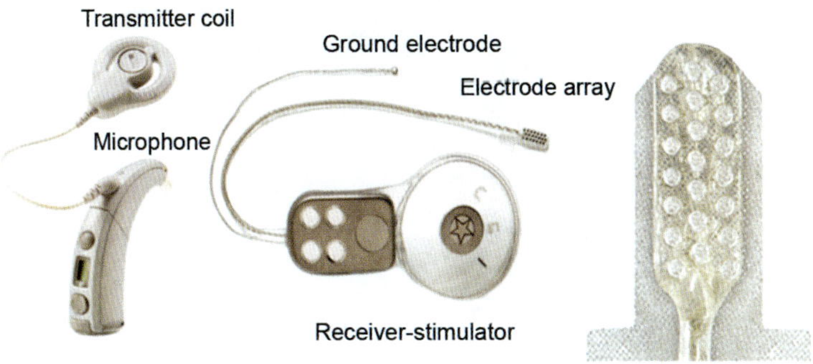

Bone anchored hearing aid (BAHA)

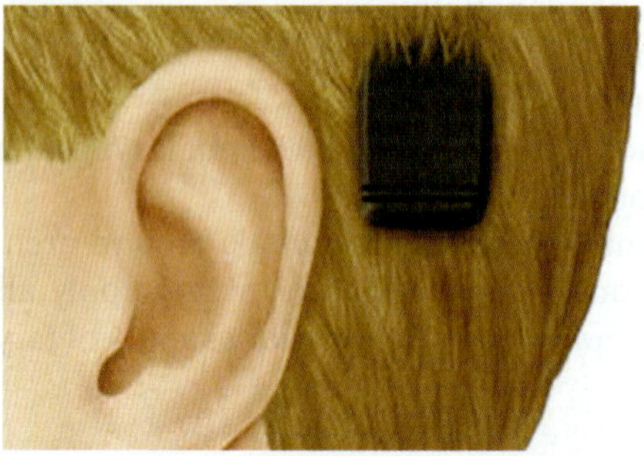

Grommet

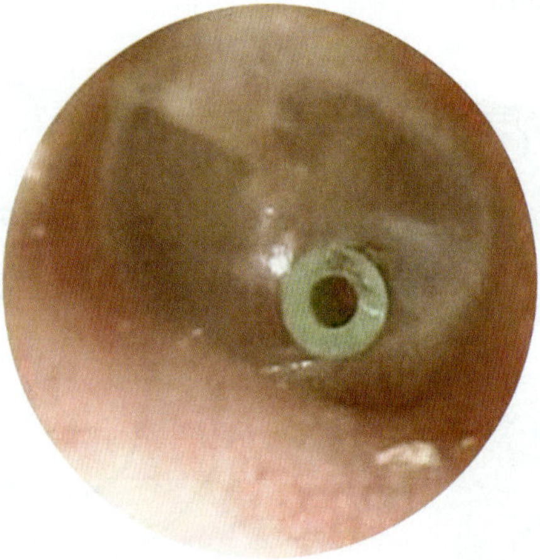

Microwick (drug introduction into inner ear)

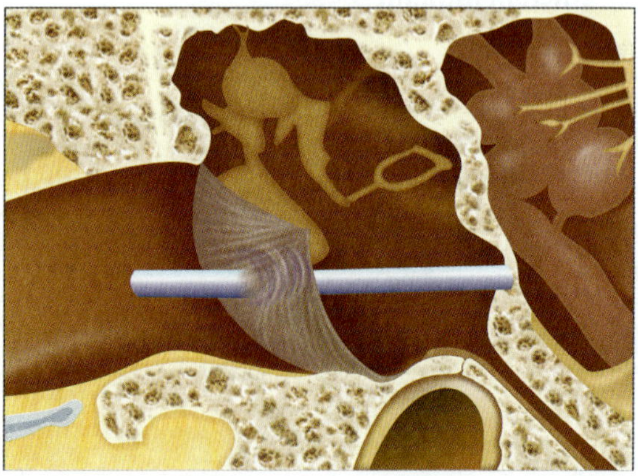

Siegel's speculum

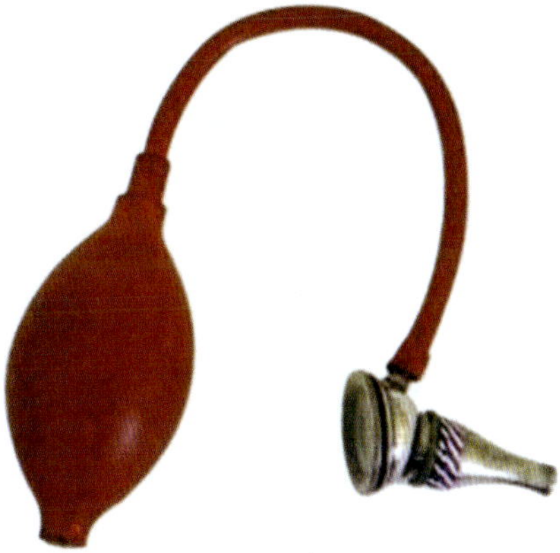

Head mirror (Focal length is ~25 cm)

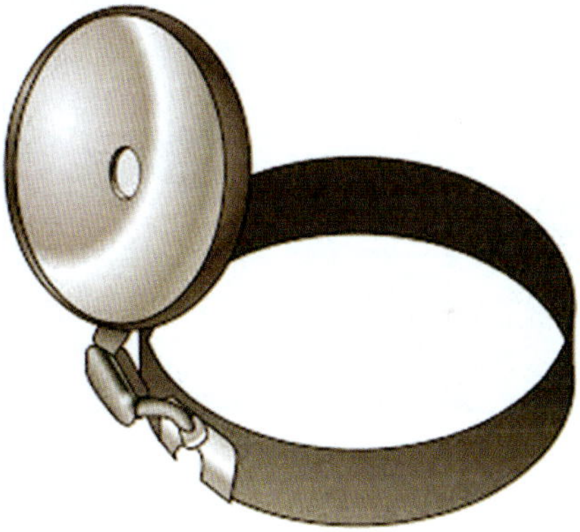

Brainstem-evoked response audiometry (BERA)

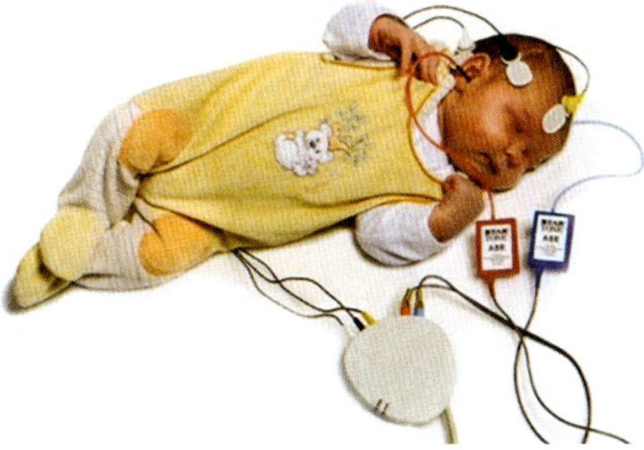

Video stroboscopy

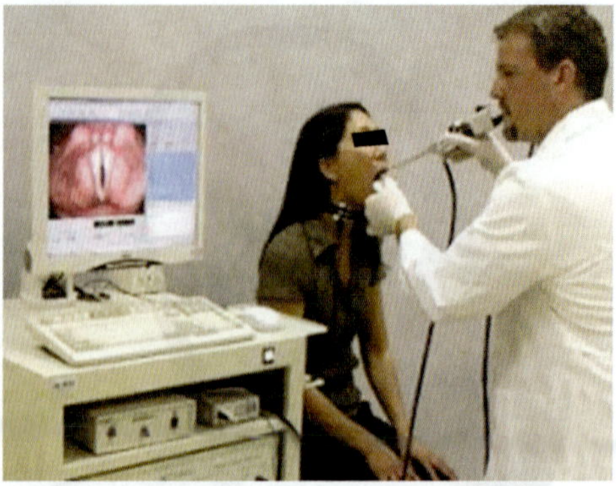

Silastic button for nasal septal perforation

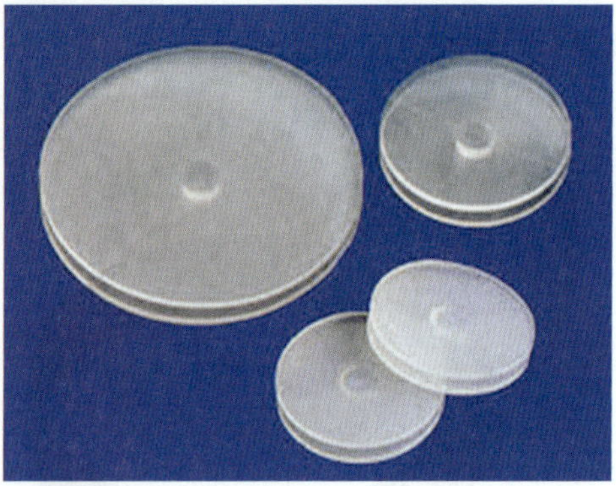

15

CHAPTER

Anesthesia

1. A patient in medical intensive care unit (ICU) who is intubated suddenly removes the endotracheal (ET) tube. What should be done next?

A. Sedate and reintubate
B. Make him sit and do physiotherapy
C. Assess the patient give bag and mask ventilation and look for spontaneous breathing
D. Give bag and mask ventillation and intubate

ANS. **C**

2. Before endotracheal intubation, preoxygenation should be done for how long?

A. 2 minutes
B. 3 minutes
C. 4 minutes
D. 5 minutes

ANS. **B**

Before intubation, preoxygenation should be done for 3 minutes.

Important topics in anesthesia

Color identification of medical gas cylinders			
Name of gas	Body	Shoulder	Pin index
Air	Gray	White and black quarter	1,5
Carbon dioxide (Concentration >7.5%)	Gray	Gray	1,6
Oxygen	Black	White	2,5

Contd...

Contd...

Carbon dioxide (Concentration >7.5%)	Gray	Gray	2,6
Nitrous oxide	Blue	Blue	3,5
Cyclopropane	Orange	Orange	3,6
Entonox (50%O_2+N_2O	Blue	Blue and white quarter	7
Helium	Brown	Brown	-
Mix of oxygen and helium (He >80.5%)	Brown	White	4,6 2,4
Nitrogon	Black	Black	1,4

Fasting required for anesthesia

1. For clear fluids: 2 hours
2. For breast milk: 3–4 hours
3. For solids: 6–8 hours

Drugs to be stopped before surgery

- Warfarin: 4–5 days prior
- LMW heparin: Therapeutic (24 hours)
- Prophylactic (12 hours)
- IV heparin: 6 hours before
- OHA/insulin: omit morning dose
- Combined OCP: 4 weeks before
- LI+: 2 days before
- Continue aspirin 75 mg (stop only for closed space surgery)
- Clopidogrel: 7 days
- Ticlopidine: 14 days
- ACEI/ARB: Omit the morning dose.

ASA scale of physical status		
ASA I	A normal healthy patient	Healthy; no smoking, no or very minimal drinking
ASA II	A patient with mild systemic disease	Smoker; more than minimal drinking; pregnancy; obesity; well-controlled diabetes, well-controlled hypertension; mild lung disease
ASA III	A patient with severe systemic disease, not incapacitating	Diabetes, poorly-controlled hypertension; distant history of myocardial infarction (MI), cerebrovascular accident (CVA), trasient ischemic attack (TIA), cardiac stent; chronic obstructive pulmonary disease (COPD), end-stage renal disease (ESRD); dialysis; active hepatitis; implanted pacemaker; ejection fraction below 40%; congenital metabolic abnormalities

ASA IV	A patient with severe systemic disease that is a constant threat to life	Recent history of MI, CVA, TIA, cardiac stent; Ongoing cardiac ischemia or severe valve dysfunction; implantable cardioverter defibrillator (ICD); ejection fraction below 25%
ASA V	A moribund patient who is not expected to survive without the operation	Ruptured abdominal or thoracic aneurism; intracranial bleed with mass effect; ischemic bowel in the face of significant cardiac pathology
ASA VI	A patient who has already been declared brain-dead and whose organs are being removed for transplant	
The addition of an 'E' indicates emergency surgery.		

Flexometallic tube for prolonged surgeries

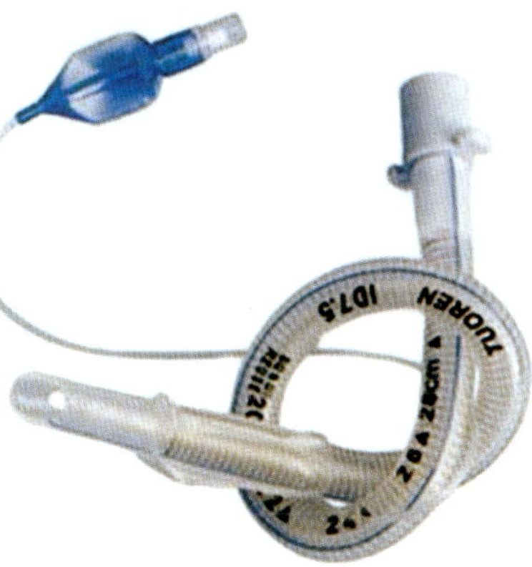

Double lumen endotracheal tube

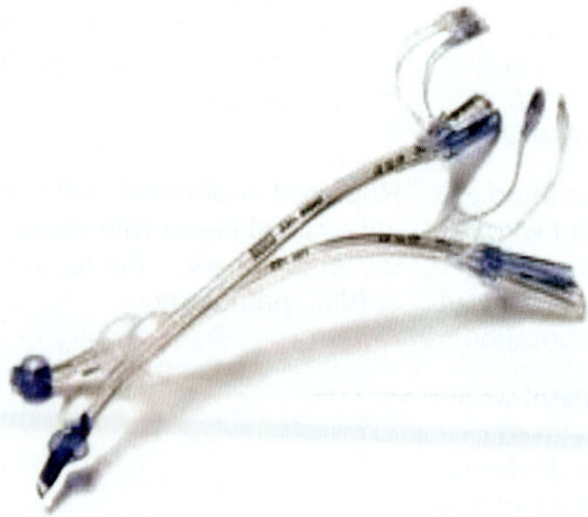

Preformed entotracheal tube

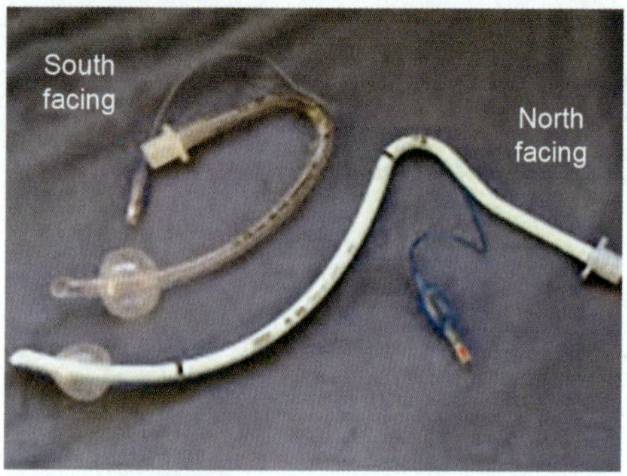

Combitube

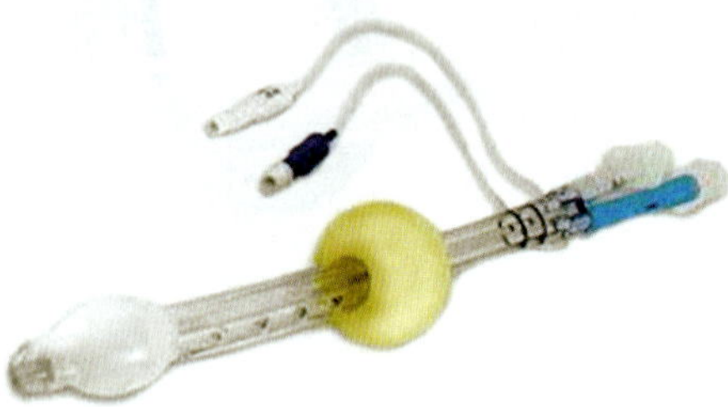

16
CHAPTER

Radiology

1. Following image shows:

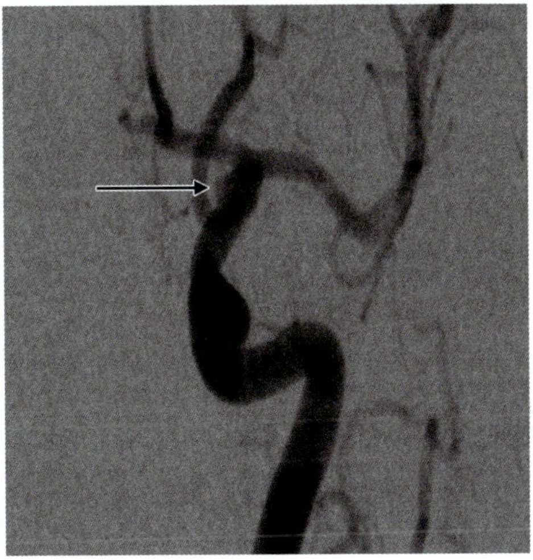

A. Angiofibroma tumor blush
B. Pseudoaneurysm at internal carotid artery
C. Aneurysm at internal maxillary artery
D. Hemangioma at the internal carotid artery

ANS. **B**

- The image shown above is a digital subtraction angiography (DSA), which shows a pseudoaneurysm at the internal carotid artery.
- Investigation of choice for aneurysm is DSA.

2. A patient presents to the emergency department of AIIMS with the most severe headache of his life. What should be done next?

A. Contrast enhanced computed tomography (CT)
B. Noncontrast CT
C. Magnetic resonance imaging (MRI)
D. Lumbar puncture (LP)

ANS. **B**

- Investigation of choice in subarachnoid hemorrhage (SAH): Noncontrast CT
- Investigation of choice in aneurysm: DSA
- Investigation which can diagnose ischemia in brain earliest: MRI (diffusion weighted imaging, within 3–30 minutes)
- First imaging investigation to be done in a patient with suspected stroke: Noncontrast CT.

3. Fluorodeoxyglucose-positron emission tomography (FDG-PET) does not detect which of the following?

A. Typical carcinoid
B. Atypical carcinoid
C. Small cell neuroendocrine tumor
D. Large cell neuroendocrine tumor

ANS. **A**

Tumors which have low metabolic rate is negative on FDG-PET. Examples of low metabolic tumors are:

1. Bronchoalveolar carcinoma
2. Carcinoid tumors.

But the question had both typical and atypical carcinoid.

Typical carcinoid has less number of mitosis than atypical carcinoid, hence, it has less metabolic rate than atypical carcinoid. So, typical carcinoid is the answer.

17

CHAPTER

Psychiatry

1. A young male patient is on 5 mg haloperidol for 4 days now he has restlessness and urge to move the legs. What is the diagnosis?

A. Akathisia B. Tardive dyskinesia
C. Rabbit syndrome D. Acute dystonia

ANS. **A**

This is an extrapyramidal side effect of typical antipsychotics.

Extrapyramidal Side Effects

Akathisia

- This is the most common EPS.
- Presents as restlessness, tapping of feet, increased pace, etc.
- Treatment is with propranolol.

Acute dystonia

- This is the earliest EPS to appear (even within hours)
- Presents as oculogyric crisis, torticolis, etc.
- Treatment is with anticholinergics (IV promethazine)

Pseudoparkinsonism

- Presents within days to weeks of starting antipsychotics
- Presents as tremor, bradykinesia, increased salivation.
- Treatment is again with anticholinergics.

Tardive dyskinesia

- Appears late during treatment.
- It is due to supersensitivity of post-synaptic dopaminergic receptors.
- Presents as abnormal movements of mouth and tongue.

- Treatment consists of changing typical antipsychotics, valbenazine/tetrabenazine.

2. A patient believes that he is the most important person in the world than anyone, so his neighbors and family is trying to harm him as they are jealous of him. His wife says otherwise and says he behaves like this recently only, before he was working as a school teacher. Diagnosis is:

A. Delusion of grandiosity
B. Delusion of persecution
C. Delusion of grandiosity and persecution
D. Delusion of grandiosity, persecution and reference

ANS. **C**

Lets analyze the question.

- The belief that I am the most important person in this world—*Delusion of grandiosity*
- The thought that others are trying to harm him because they are jealous—*Delusion of persecution*
- The catch in the question is whether there is delusion of reference. Delusion of reference is, thought that things or places are related to him.

3. An IT employee after taking up the job is feeling guilty, hopeless and not able to concentrate on work. His symptoms started 3 years back when he entered college. Likely diagnosis?

A. Depressive disorder
B. Dysthymia
C. Adjustment disorder
D. Cyclothymia

ANS. **B**

Symptoms of hopelessness, guilt and loss of concentration for more than 2 years is called dysthymia.

4. Basis of reliability of information of patient provided by informants depend on all *except:*

A. Biological relationship
B. Educational status
C. Observational skill
D. Duration of stay with patient

ANS. **C**

Basis of reliablity of patient history by informants depends upon:

- Age
- Sex

- Educational status
- Marital status
- History of physical illness
- Duration of stay with patient
- Relationship with patient.

Observational skill is not a basis of reliablity in history taking, moreover it is not measurable also.

5. A young patient was admitted to hospital with acute psychosis. He wakes up and asks for his wife who was there in the same room in same area. Upon seeing her he started beating her thinking it was the nurse who was masqeurading as his wife. He also said she was the same nurse who gave him wrong medication 2 days back as well to make him ill, because she wanted to harm him, but it was his wife who gave wrong medicine. Diagnosis?

A. Capgras syndrome B. Fregoli syndrome
C. Othello D. Cotard syndrome

ANS. **A**

- Here, the nurse (prosecutor) has taken the form of a family member (wife)—this phenomenon is called Capgras syndrome.
- Delusion in Capgras syndrome is the belief that the persecutor has taken the form of family members.
- When the persecutor is a family member (When wife wants to kill him, she takes the form of nurse as a disguise to kill him)—this is Fregoli syndrome

6. Which of the following is the test for immediate memory?

A. Serial (100-7) subtraction test up to 5 steps
B. Digit span forward up to 7 digits with 2 steps allowed
C. Digit span backward up to 7 digits with 2 steps allowed
D. Serial 20-1 subtraction test up to 5 steps.

ANS. **A**

Memory can be:

- Immediate
- Recent
- Remote

Tests for immediate memory:

- Digit span test

- Serial (100-7) subtraction test
- Days of week backward
- Spell world backwards
- (20-3) test.

Catch points at options

- In digit span test, we have to spell at 1 digit/second
- Test is stopped when there is 2 successive failures (Hence, option B and C are wrong).

Criteria for duration of diagnosis of each psychiatric disorder

	ICD-10	*DSM 5*
Schizophrenia	1 month	6 months
Dementia	6 months	6 months
Depression	2-weeks	2 weeks
Mania	1 week	1 week
PTSD	1 month	1 month
Cyclothymia/Dysthymia	2 years	2 years

Abbreviations: PTSD, post-traumatic stress disorder

Clusters of personality disorder (PD)

Cluster A (odd and eccentric)	• Paranoid PD • Schizoid PD • Schizotypal PD
Cluster B (dramatic, emotional and erratic)	• Antisocial PD • Histrionic PD • Narcissistic PD • Borderline PD
Cluster C (anxious and fearful)	• Anxious (avoidant) PD • Dependent PD • Anankastic (obsessive and compulsive) PD

Phases of sexual cycle

Stage of desire

- Excess desire in males: Satyriasis
- Excess desire in females: Nymphomania.

Stage of arousal/excitement

- This is the longest phase.
- This stage is impaired in erectile dysfunction.

Stage of orgasm (ejaculation)
- This is the shortest phase.
- This phase is impaired in premature ejaculation.

Phase of resolution
This phase includes post-coital dysphoria.

Psychotherapy

Supportive psychotherapy: Psychotherapy of choice for adjustment disorder.

Re-educative psychotherapy:
- This includes cognitive behavior therapy (CBT)
- CBT is the psychotherapy of choice in:
  - Depression
  - Obsessive-compulsive disorder (OCD)
  - Post-traumatic stress disorder (PTSD)

Other important psychotherapy
- Phobia: Systemic desensitization
- Paraphilia: Aversion
- Nocturnal eneuresis: Bed alarm
- PTSD: EMDR (eye movement desensitisation and reprocessing)
- PTSD: Crisis intervention.

Defense mechanisms

Repression is the mother of all defense mechanism.

Mature defense mechanism
- Sublimation
- Anticipation
- Humor
- Altruism
- Supression.

Defense mechanism in OCD
- Undoing
- Reaction formation
- Regression

Defense mechanism in substance use
- Denial
- Rationalization

Personality disorders
- Schizotypal: Magical thinking
- Borderline: Emotionally unstable (suicidal tendencies).

- Hystrionic: Attention seeking
- Narcissistic: Self love
- Antisocial: Break rules
- OCPD/anankistic: Perfectionist.

Neurotransmitters in psychiatric disorders

Schizophrenia
- Dopamine and 5-HT increase
- ACh (acetylcholine), glutamate, GABA, norepinephrine decreases.

Depression
- ACh and glutamate increases
- Dopamine, 5-HT, norepinephrine, GABA (gamma-aminobutyric acid) decreases.

Dementia
- ACh decreases
- Glutamate increases.

Suicide
- 5 HT decreases.

Delirium
- ACh decreases.

Schizophrenia—good prognosis

- Late onset
- Precipitating factors +
- Acute onset
- Good premorbid personality
- Married
- Family history of mood disorders
- Good support systems
- Positive symptoms.

18

CHAPTER

Pediatrics

1. A term newborn presented with serum bilirubin of 18 mg/dL on the third day of life. Which of the following should be done next?

A. Continue breastfeeding and give phototherapy
B. Give exchange transfusion
C. Stop breastfeeding and give phototherapy
D. Observe as it is physiological

ANS. A

Points to be note in neonatal hyperbilirubinemia

1. Never stop breastfeeding
2. For serum bilirubin >10 mg/dL at 24 hours—do phototherapy
3. For serum bilirubin >13 mg/dL at 48 hours—do partial exchange transfusion
4. For serum bilirubin >15 mg/dL at 72 hours—do phototherapy
5. For serum bilirubin >18 mg/dL at 96 hours—do phototherapy

2. Apgar stands for: *(Asked twice in exam)*

A. Attitude pulse grimace activity respiratory effort
B. Attitude pulse grimace appearance respiratory effort
C. Appearance pulse grimace activity respiratory effort
D. Appearance pulse grimace attitude respiratory effort

ANS. C

Apgar scoring system

	0 Points	1 Points	2 Points	Points totaled
Activity (muscle tone)	Absent	Arms and legs flexed	Active movement	
Pulse	Absent	Below 100 bpm	Over 100 bpm	
Grimace (reflex irritability)	Flaccid	Some flexion of extremities	Active motion (sneeze, cough, pull away)	
Appearance (skin color)	Blue, pale	Body pink, Extremities blue	Completely pink	
Respiration	Absent	Slow, irregular	Vigorous cry	

Severely depressed	0–3
Moderately depressd	4–6
Excellent condition	7–10

3. Failure to do which of the following tasks indicates developmental delay in a 3-year-old?

A. Spoon feeding
B. Skipping
C. Draw a square
D. Climb alternate steps downwards

ANS. **A**

- Spoon feeding: 18 months
- Skipping: 5 years
- Climbs alternate step downstairs: 4 years

Upper limit of age for attainment of milestones

- Visual fixation: 2 months
- Vocalization: 6 months
- Sitting without support: 10 months
- Standing with assistance: 12 months
- Hands and knee crawling: 14 months
- Standing alone: 17 months
- Walking alone: 18 months
- Single words: 18 months
- Imaginative play: 3 years.

19
CHAPTER

Medicine

1. The following ECG shows:

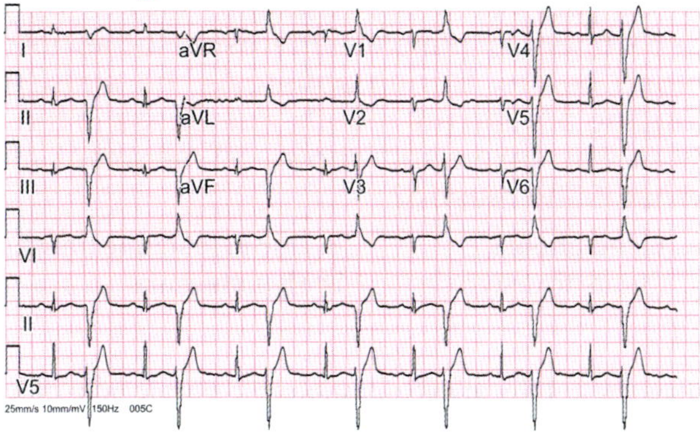

A. Ventricular bigemini B. P. pulmonale

C. Electrical alternans D. Wrong calibration

ANS. **A**

This was not the exact ECG asked. But the options were the same.

P. pulmonale

Criteria: (A) >2.5 mm in inferior leads (2, 3, AVF)

(B) >1.5 mm in V1 and V2

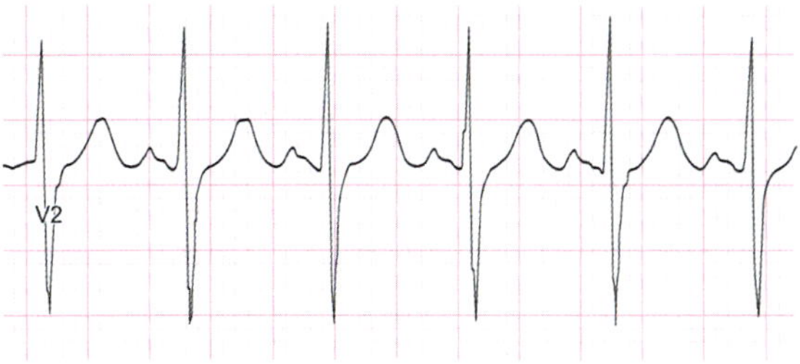

Electrical alternans

1. Consecutive normally conducted QRS complexes in height
2. Seen in pericardial effusion.

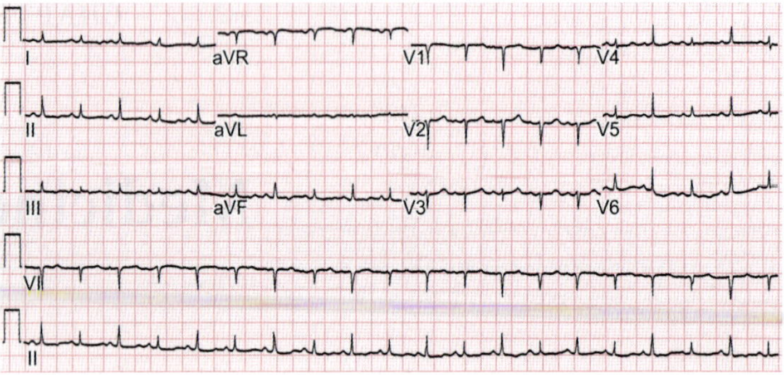

2. A 30-year-old male attends blood transfusion department for platelet apheresis. He has not donated blood before. During apheresis, he suddenly feels tingling around the mouth, numbness in the arm. An ECG was taken and shows ST segment elevation. What is the reason?

A. Blood phobia
B. Due to first time transfusion
C. Citrate toxicity
D. Hypothermia

ANS. **C**

The diagnosis of the above question is hypocalcemia due to excess citrate producing symptoms of hypocalcemic tetany.

ECG—characteristics of hypocalcemia

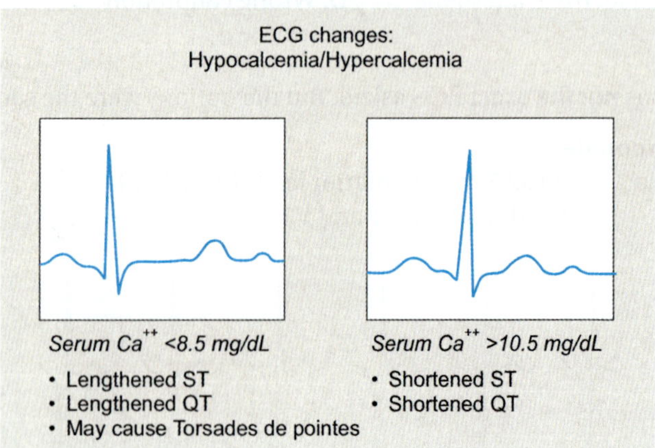

3. A 2-year-old male has developmental delay kinke hair and weak muscle tone. What is the diagnosis?

A. Wilson's disease B. Menkes disease
C. Zinc deficiency D. Cerebral palsy

ANS. **B**

Menkes disease, also known as **Menkes syndrome**, is an X-linked recessive disorder that affects copper levels in the body, leading to copper deficiency (ATB 7A gene on chromosome 13).

Signs and symptoms of this disorder include:

1. Weak muscle tone (hypotonia)
2. Sagging facial features
3. Seizures
4. Intellectual disability and developmental delay
5. Brittle hair
6. Metaphyseal widening.

Menkes disease

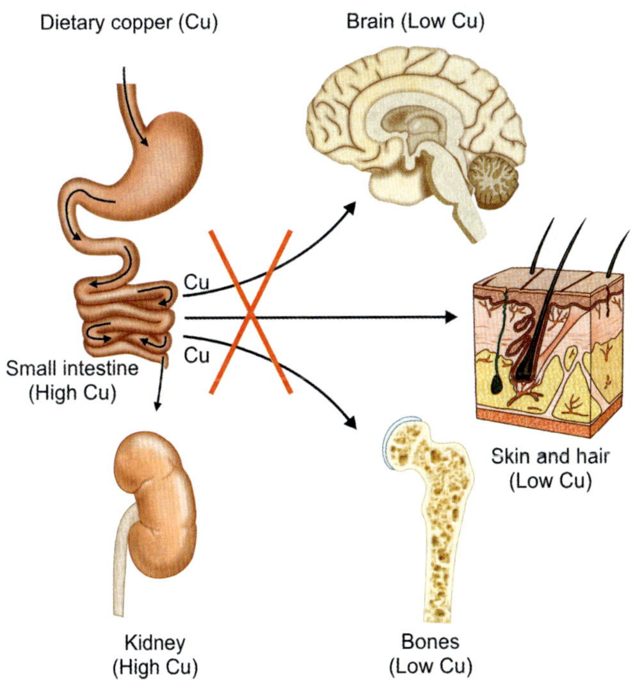

Image of zinc deficiency (acrodermatitis enteropathica)

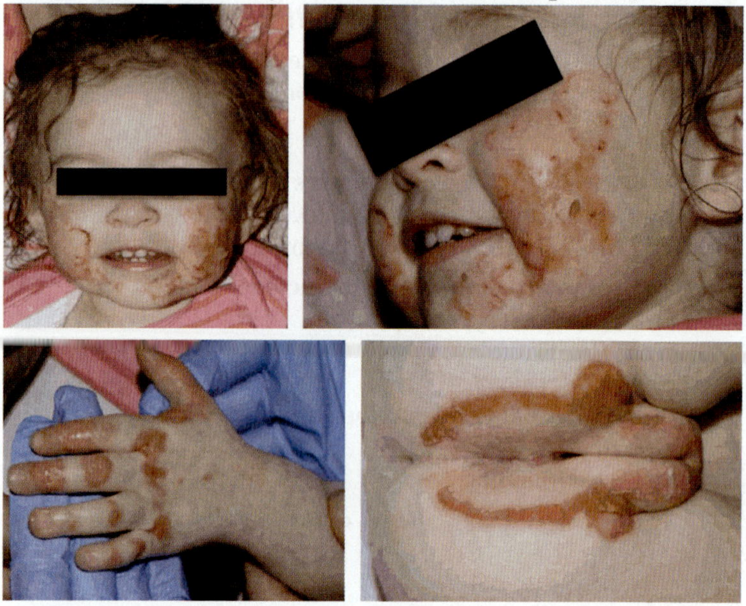

4. An intensive care unit (ICU) nurse is doing tracheostomy suction for a patient. How long does she do suction at a time?

A. 30 seconds
B. 60 seconds
C. 10–15 seconds
D. 2 minutes

ANS. **C**

If we leave the suctioning catheter for more than 15 seconds, patient will not be able to breathe well and this may lead to hypoxia.

Additional points in tracheostomy suctioning:

1. If the patient has an acute spinal cord injury, we must not insert the catheter more than 1–2 cm beyond the end of the tracheostomy tube as there is danger of vagus nerve overstimulation causing bradycardia and cardiac arrest.
2. Do not reintroduce catheter at any point as this will cause cross infection.
3. Note the color, consistency, and volume of secretions
4. To prevent hypoxia, reduce the trauma and optimize the number of times a patient will need suctioning.

5. The image shown below is from a patient who is suffering from:

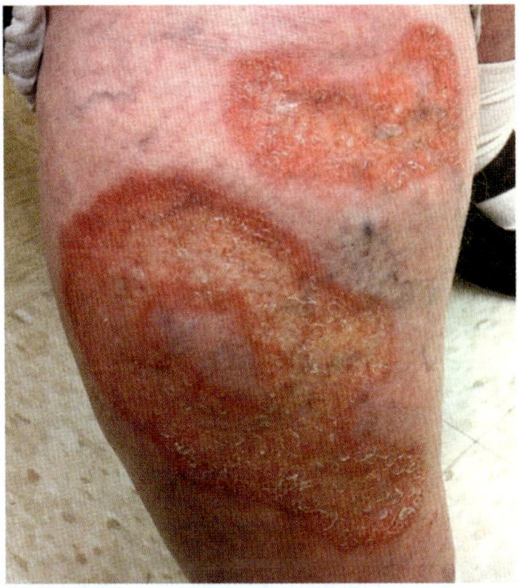

A. Sarcoidosis B. Diabetes
C. Lymes disease D. Graves disease

ANS. **B**

The image shows necrobiosis lipoidica, a classical skin change seen in diabetes. Other skin changes in diabetes are:

1. Diabetic rubeosis

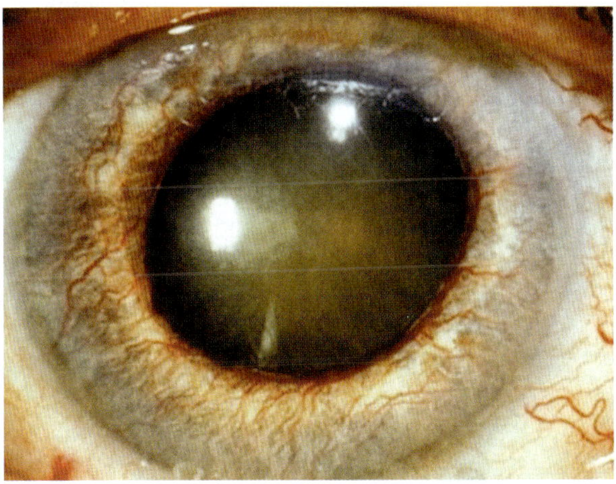

2. Spotted leg syndrome

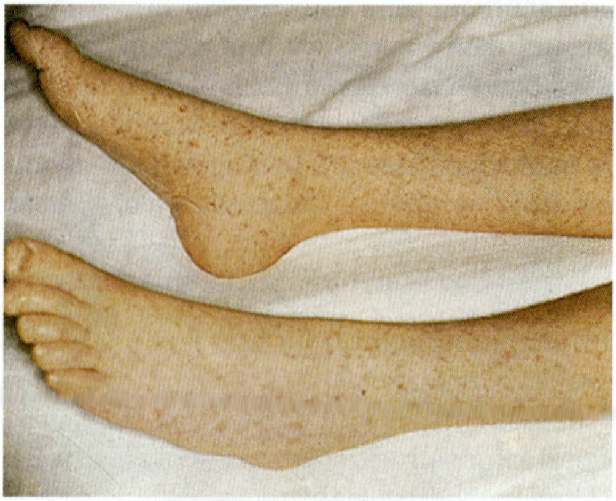

3. Scleredema diabeticorum

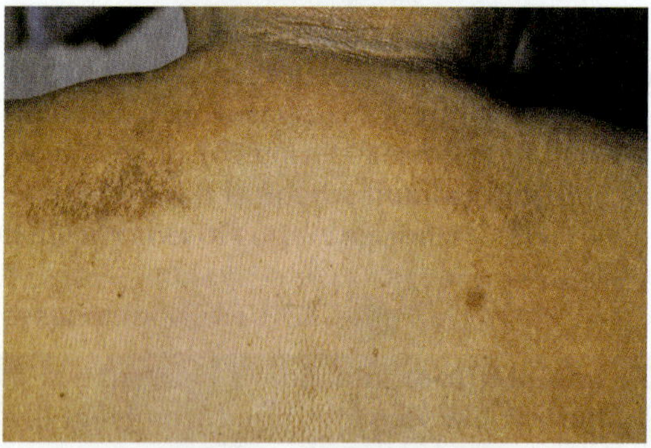

4. Diagonal earlobe crease

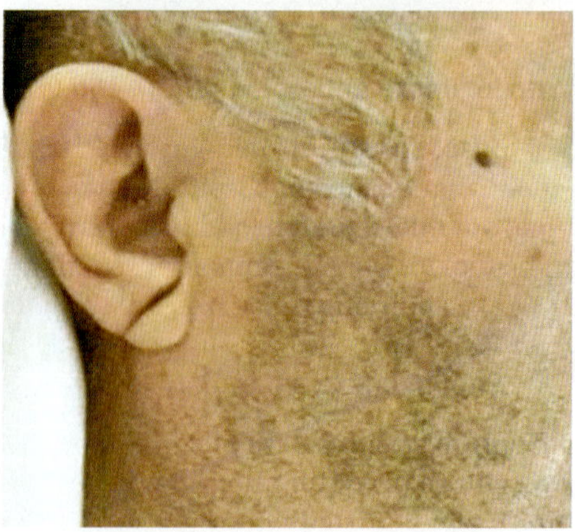

6. In a patient with mitral stenosis, disappearance of Loud S1 is associated with all *except*:

A. Calcified valve
B. Aortic regurgitation
C. Heart block
D. Mild mitral stenosis

ANS. **D**

Conditions associated with dulling of S1 (disappearance of loud S1) in patient with mitral stenosis:

1. Calcified mitral valve
2. Aortic regurgitation (AR)
3. Mitral regurgitation (MR)

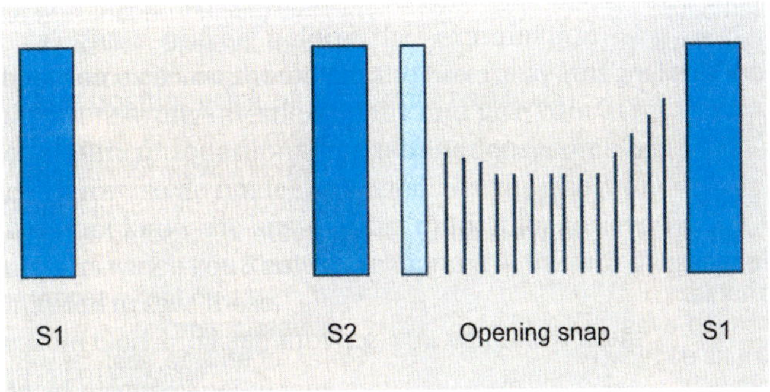

Absence of presystolic accentuation in mitral stenosis:

1. Atrial fibrillation
2. Presence of MR
3. Flabby left atrium
4. Atrial septal defect (ASD)
5. After surgery
6. Junctional rhythm.

7. You and your friend goes for a picnic to a hilly area. He has 5 to 6 episodes of loose stools. There is no fever, tachycardia or no other signs of dehydration. What should you do next?

A. Start a course of oral ofloxacin and onidazole
B. Give ORS solution with water
C. Take him to a nearby hospital
D. Start intravenous (IV) fluids

ANS. **B**

Classification of diarrhea based on severity in children and management.

Signs	*Classify as*	*Identify treatment (Urgent pre-referral treatment are in bold print)*
Two of the following signs: • Lethargic or unconscious • Sunken eyes • Not able to drink or drinking poorly • Skin pinch goes back very slowly	**Severe dehydration**	• If child has no other severe classification Give fluid of severe dehydration (Plan C) OR If child also has another severe classification Refer urgently to hospital with mother giving frequent sips of ORS on the way. Advise the mother to continue breastfeeding • If child is 2 years or older, and there is cholera in your area, give antibiotic for cholera.
Two of the following signs: • Restless, irritable • Sunken eyes • Drinks eagerly, thirsty • Skin pinch goes back slowly.	**Some dehydration**	• Give fluid, zinc supplements and food for some dehydration (Plan B) • *If child also has a severe classification:* Refer urgently to hospital with mother giving frequent sips of ORS on the way. Advise the mother to continue breastfeeding • Advise mother when to return immediately • Follow-up in 5 days if not improving • If confirmed/symptomatic HIV, follow-up in 2 days if not improving
• Not enough signs to classify as some or severe dehydration	**No dehydration**	• Give fluid, zinc supplements and food to treat diarrhea at home (Plan A) • Advise mother when to return immediately • *Follow-up in 5 days if not improving* • If confirmed/symptomatic HIV, follow-up in 2 days if not improving

8. Serum ascites albumin gradient less than 1.1 is seen in all of the following *except*:

A. Nephrotic syndrome B. Tuberculosis
C. Malignancy D. Congestive cardiac failure

ANS. **D**

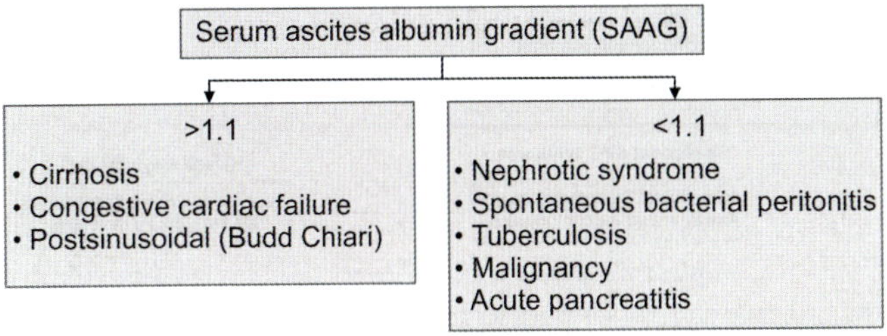

All transudates have SAAG >1.1 Except nephrotic syndrome which has SAAG <1.1

9. Metabolic acidosis with normal anion gap is seen all of the following conditions *except*:

A. Salicylic acid poisoning B. Diarrhea
C. Renal tubular acidosis D. Chronic pancreatitis

ANS. **A**

Metabolic acidosis with normal anion gap:
1. Renal tubular acidosis
2. Diarrhea
3. Chronic pancreatitis
4. Ureterosigmoidostomy
5. Villous adenoma
6. Hydrogen chloride poisoning

Metabolic acidosis with increased anion gap:
1. Diabetic ketoacidosis
2. Lactic acidosis
3. Renal failure
4. Salicylate poisoning
5. Methanol poisoning
6. Paraldehyde poisoning
7. Ethylene glycol poisoning

10. A 45-year-old man presents with exertional dyspnea and pitting pedal edema. His neck veins are dilated. A diagnosis of superior vena cava (SVC) syndrome is made. What will you do next?

A. Do total blood count and peripheral smear
B. Do a CT chest
C. Start cyclophosphamide
D. Start radiotherapy

ANS. **B**

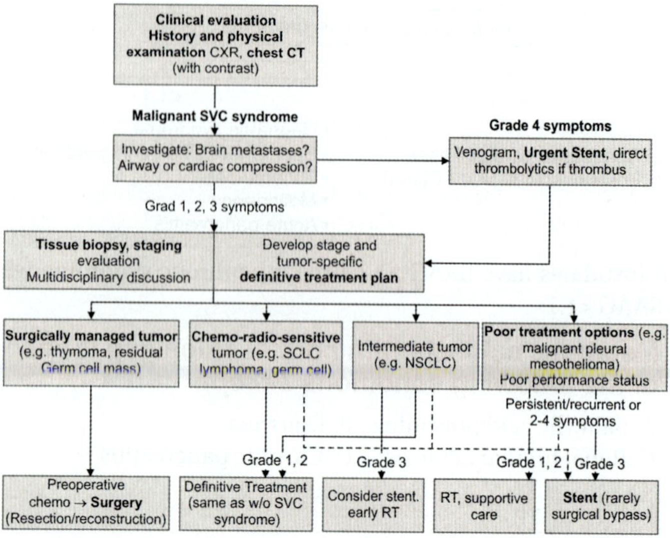

This shows an approach to a case of SVC syndrome which clearly says that first step is CT chest with contrast. This helps us to arrive at a cause for SVC syndrome and treat accordingly.

Various causes of SVC syndrome are:

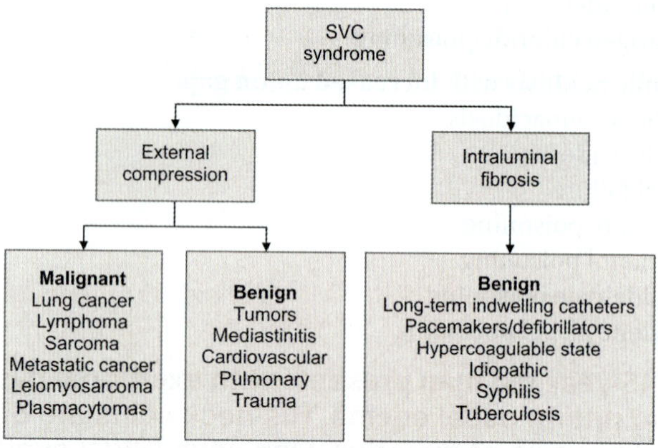

11. During a routine follow-up of a hypertensive patient, an intern noticed that the BP on right arm was 150/100 and on the left arm was 90/60. On examination, there was a mid-diastolic murmur on the second aortic area. Which of the following conditions is least likely the cause of his hypertension?

A. Coarctation of aorta
B. Takayasu arteritis
C. Aortic dissection
D. Supravalvular aortic stenosis

ANS. **D**

This question may look complicated, but the catch is mid-diastolic murmur.

Coarctation of aorta, Takayasu and aortic dissection can cause mid-diastolic murmur but aortic stenosis causes systolic murmur, hence, it is least likely diagnosis in this case.

Causes of anisosphygmia (Difference in pulse volume on identical vessels of both sides)

1. Coarctation of aorta
2. Takayasu's disease
3. Subclavian steal syndrome

12. The following images show which clinical condition?

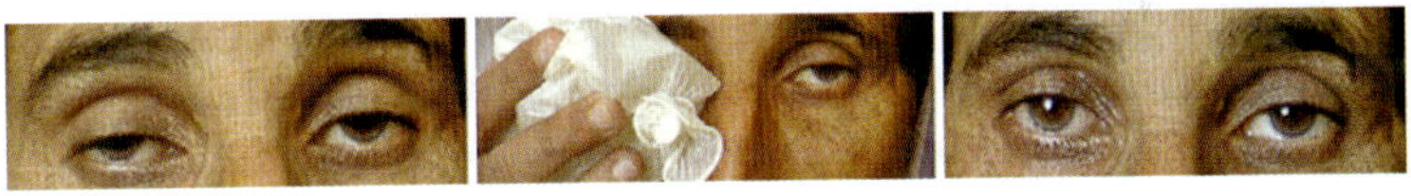

Fig. 1: Bilateral ptosis (More marked in right eye)

Fig. 2: Ice pack application on right eye

Fig. 3: Improvement in ptosis of right eye after ice pack application

A. Tolosa-Hunt syndrome
B. Myasthenia gravis
C. Trigeminal neuralgia
D. Multiple sclerosis

ANS. **B**

The image shows the ice pack test used for the diagnosis of myasthenia gravis.

Pathogenesis of myasthenia gravis

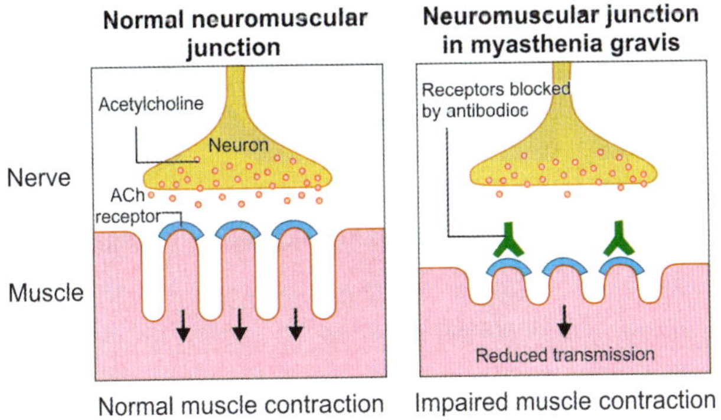

Important points in myasthenia gravis

1. *Most sensitive test:* EMG (decremental response)
2. *Most specific test:* Antibody against ACh esterase antibody
3. *Treatment of myasthenic crisis:* Plasmapheresis and IVIG
4. *Indications for thymectomy in MG:*
   a. Anti-MuSK negative
   b. Presence of thymoma or thymic hyperplasia
5. *Contraindications for thymectomy:*
   a. Age <15 years and >55 years
   b. Anti MuSK positive
   c. Generalized MG

Osserman classification of myasthenia gravis (MG)

1. Occular MG
2. Generalized MG
3. Bulbar weakness
4. Respiratory weakness/crisis

13. For the evaluation of a patient with headache and fever, a CSF analysis was done and it revealed.

Cell count: 40 lymphocytes
CSF protein: 55
CSF glucose: 64
Opening pressure: 190 mm Hg

What is the most likely diagnosis?

A. Tuberculosis B. Coxsackie
C. *N. meningitidis* D. *Cryptococcus*

ANS. **B**

Test	*Appearance*	*Pressure*	*WBC/ μL*	*Protein mg/dL*	*Glucose mg/dL*	*Chloride*
Normal CSF	Clear	90–180 mm	0–8 lymph	15–45	50–80	115–130 mEq/L
Acute bacterial meningitis	Turbid	Increased	1000–10000	100–500	<40	Decreased
Viral meningitis	Clear	Normal to moderate increase	5–300, rarely >1000	Normal to mild increased	Normal	Normal

Contd...

Contd...

Tubercular meningitis	Slightly opaque cobweb formation	Increase/ decreased, spinal block	100–600 mixed or lymph	50–300 due to spinal block	Decreased	Decreased
Fungal meningitis	Clear	Increased	40–400 mixed	50–300	Decreased	Decreased
Acute syphilitic	Clear	Increased	About 500 lymph	Increased but < 100	Normal	Decreased

14. Hepatitis B remains in latent period for a long time but still there is increased risk of HCC, what is the cause of this transformation?

A. Inability to induce inflammation to remove organism
B. High level of transaminase
C. High rate of proliferation of hepatocyte
D. Risk of integration of viral DNA with host DNA.

ANS. **D**

Let us analyze this question by looking at each option.

Option A is a correct statement, but inability to induce inflammation is not the cause for transformation into hepatocellular carcinoma.

Option B is not definitely the cause for HCC as elevated transaminases does not have anything to do with HCC.

Option C is not correct as in latent period, there is no proliferation of hepatocytes.

Option D is the answer and integration of viral DNA with host DNA causes transformation into HCC.

20

CHAPTER

Emergency Medicine

1. A person suddenly fell unconscious and he is unresponsive. You call for help. By the time help arrives you should:

A. Start C-reactive protein
B. Check for pulse
C. Give defibrillation
D. Check for breathing and give mouth to mouth respiration

ANS. **B**

2. A patient was brought to the emergency medicine department of AIIMS with history of renal tubular acidosis (RTA). He had eye movement on response to pain, was speaking inappropriate sentence, and moved all limbs spontaneously. What is his Glasgow coma scale (GCS) score?

A. 13
B. 8
C. 10
D. 11

ANS. **D**

3. A 25-year-old man presented to the emergency medicine department with acute onset sharp pain and dyspnea. His chest X-ray (CXR) is given here. What is the diagnosis?

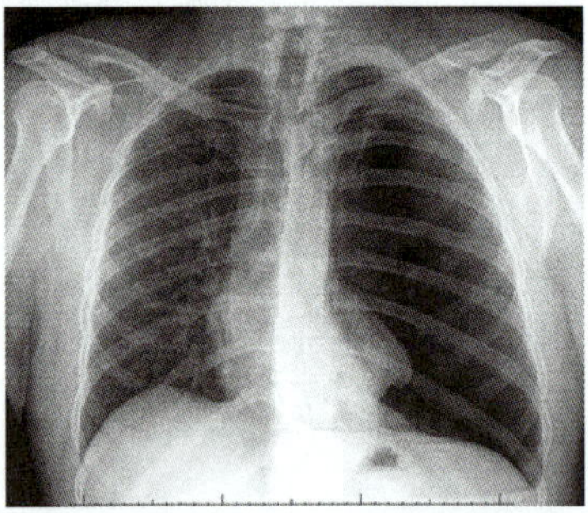

A. Pleural effusion
B. Pulmonry embolism

C. Hydropneumothorax
D. Spontaneous pneumothorax

ANS. **D**

4. A patient comes to the emergency medicine department with acute onset of palpitation. His systolic BP was 96 mm Hg. His ECG shows narrow complex tachycardia. Which of the following should be done next?

A. Intravenous adenosine
B. Intravenous diltiazem
C. Defibrillation
D. Carotid body massage

ANS. **A**

5. A patient with history of weakness of one side was brought to AIIMS emergency medicine department with altered sensorium. A CT was taken, and showed the following. What should be done next?

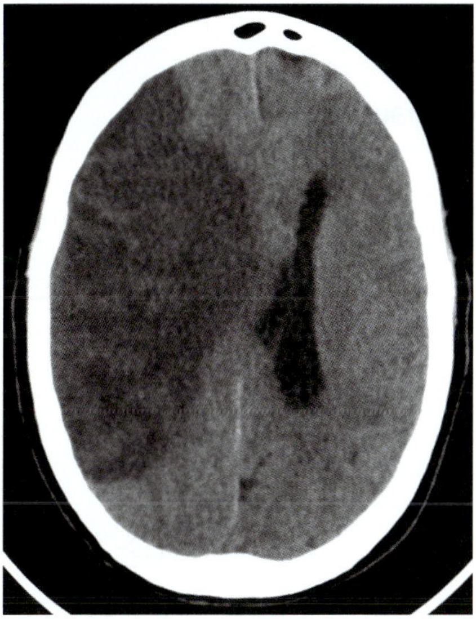

A. Decompressive craniotomy
B. Intravenous mannitol
C. Observe and follow-up
D. Aspirin

ANS. **B**

6. For the transport of traumatized and conscious patient all of the following are done *except*:

A. On a hard board with head/spine stabilized
B. In a lateral lying position
C. Talk to patient while he is on board
D. Rolling without moving the spine

ANS. **B**

Prevention of C-spine injury

1. Prevent further injury by C-spine control
2. Immobilize the patient on to a hard background
3. Transportation of patient by emergency medical team.

7. In triage of school bus accident of children, which one will you attend first and give priority?

A. Airway obstruction of child
B. Boy in shock
C. Flair chest child
D. Severe head injury

ANS. **A**

Evaluation of a trauma victim

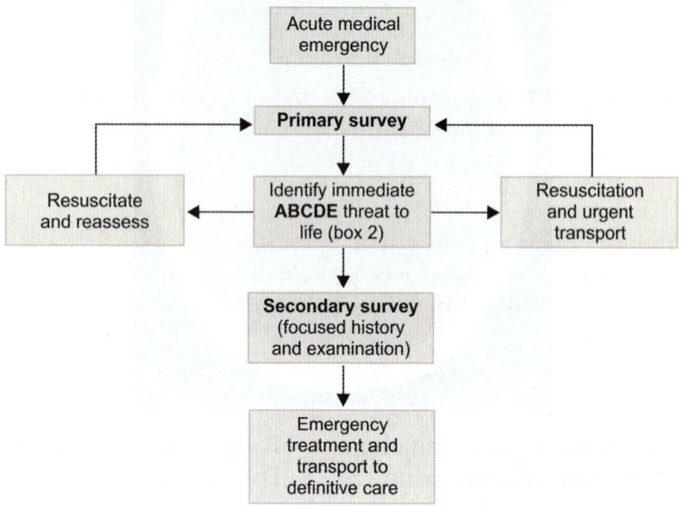

Primary survey in trauma

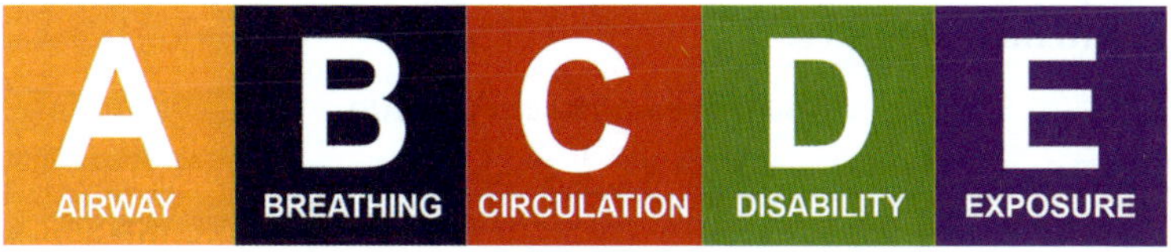

Focused history and physical examination (secondary survey)

The focused history and physical examination includes a physical examination that focuses on a specific injury or medical complaint, or it may be a rapid examination of the entire body.

It also includes obtaining a patient history and vital signs.

Patient history: A patient history includes any information relating to the current complaint or condition, as well as past medical problems that could be related. Utilize bystanders/family... when needed.

Acronym to obtain a patient's history:
S: Signs/symptoms
A: Allergies
M: Medications
P: Pertinent past medical history
L: Last oral intake
E: Events leading to the illness or injury

Rapid assessment: This a quick, less detailed head-to-toe assessment of the most critical patients.

Focused assessment: This is an examination conducted on stable patients. It focuses on a specific injury or medical complaint.

Vital signs: This include pulse, respirations, skin signs, pupils, and blood pressure. This may include documenting the oxygen saturation level (this is highly useful when dealing with chemical agent exposure).

Pulse: Assess for rate, rhythm, and strength.

Respiration: Assess for rate, depth, sound, and ease of breathing.

Skin signs: Assess for color, temperature, and moisture.

Pupils: Check pupils for size, equality, and reaction to light. Constricted pupils in a mass casualty event are highly suggestive of nerve agent/organophosphate toxicity.

Head-to toe examination of a trauma patient with significant MOI—The physical examination of the patient should take not more than **two to three minutes.**

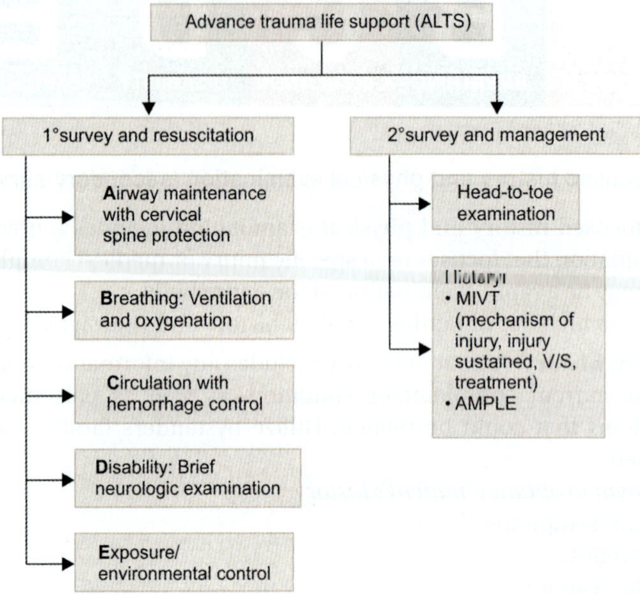

Chain of survival

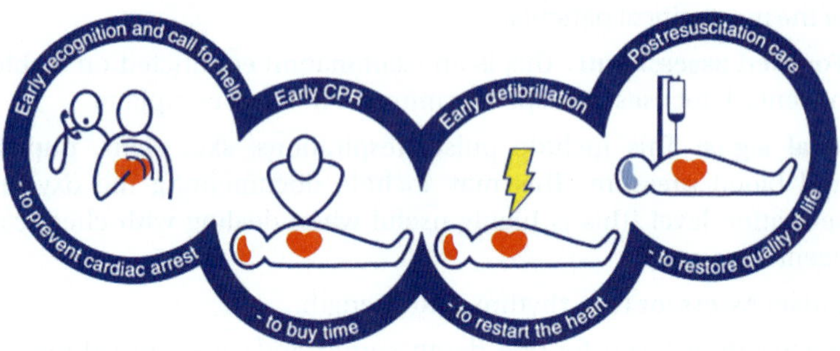

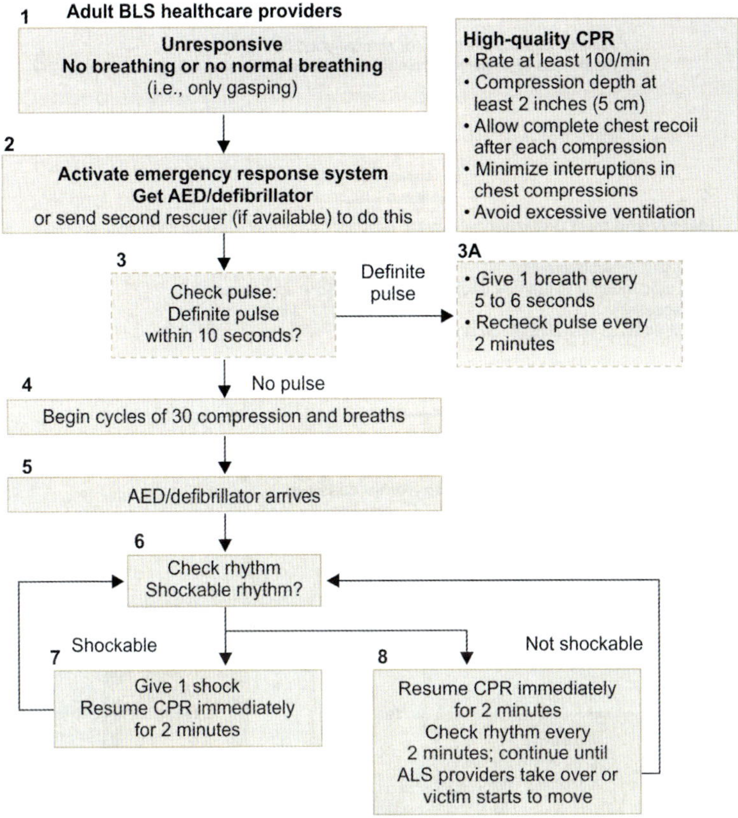

Note: The boxes bordered with dashed lines are performed by healthcare providers and not by lay rescuers

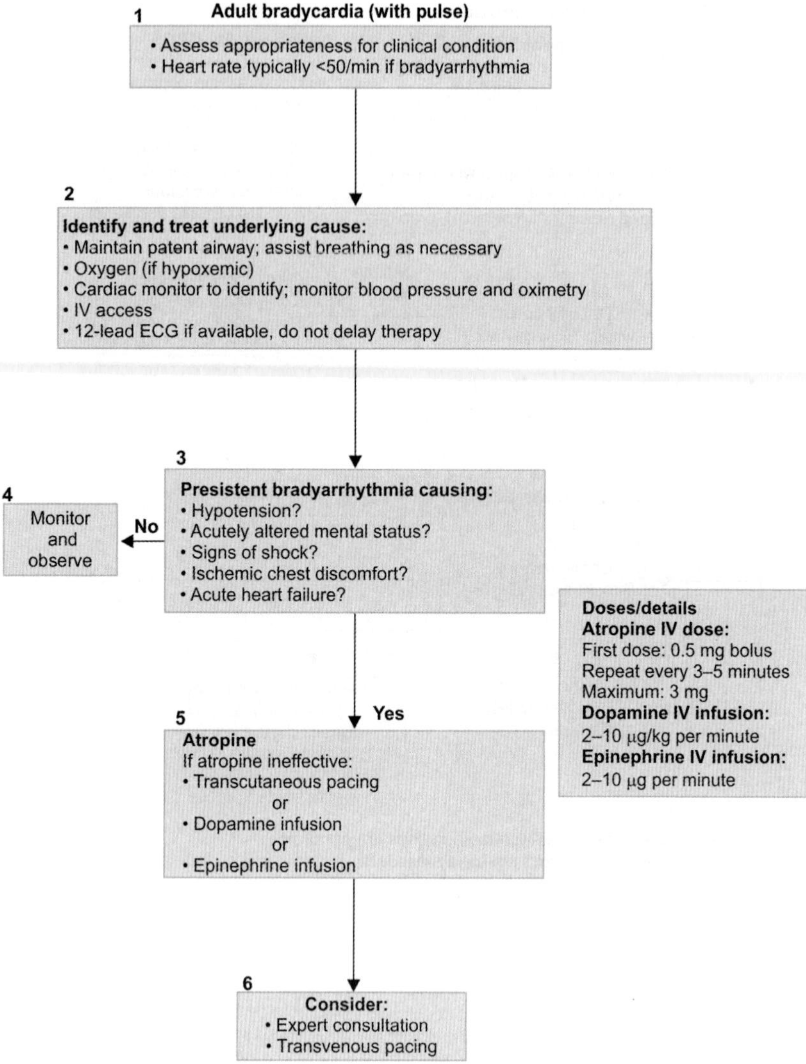
1 Adult bradycardia (with pulse)
• Assess appropriateness for clinical condition
• Heart rate typically <50/min if bradyarrhythmia
2
Identify and treat underlying cause:
• Maintain patent airway; assist breathing as necessary
• Oxygen (if hypoxemic)
• Cardiac monitor to identify; monitor blood pressure and oximetry
• IV access
• 12-lead ECG if available, do not delay therapy
3
Presistent bradyarrhythmia causing:
• Hypotension?
• Acutely altered mental status?
• Signs of shock?
• Ischemic chest discomfort?
• Acute heart failure?
No
4
Monitor and observe
Yes
5
Atropine
If atropine ineffective:
• Transcutaneous pacing
or
• Dopamine infusion
or
• Epinephrine infusion
6
Consider:
• Expert consultation
• Transvenous pacing
Doses/details
Atropine IV dose:
First dose: 0.5 mg bolus
Repeat every 3–5 minutes
Maximum: 3 mg
Dopamine IV infusion:
2–10 μg/kg per minute
Epinephrine IV infusion:
2–10 μg per minute

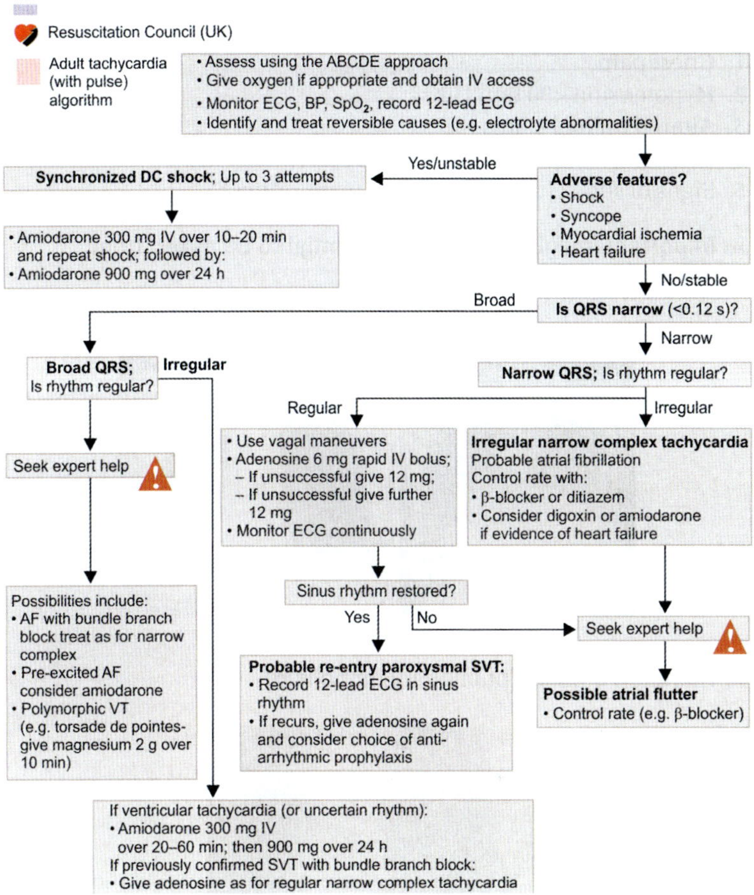

To simplify

- *Treatment of unstable tachycardia:* Synchronized DC version
- *Treatment of stable tachycardia:* Drugs and carotid massage
- *Treatment of unstable bradycardia:* Transcutaneous pacing/ medical pacing (atropine 0.5 mg (up to 3 mg) or injection adrenaline (2–20 µg/kg/min) or injection dopamine (2–20 µg/kg/min)
- *Treatment of stable bradycardia:* Expert consultation for identifying cause.

How to say a patient is stable or not (look for CHAPS)

1. **C**hest pain
2. **H**ypotension <90 mm Hg
3. **A**ltered mental status
4. **P**ulmonary signs of cardiac failure (crepitations)
5. **S**igns of shock (cold and clammy extremities)

Important imaging questions potential to be asked from emergencies

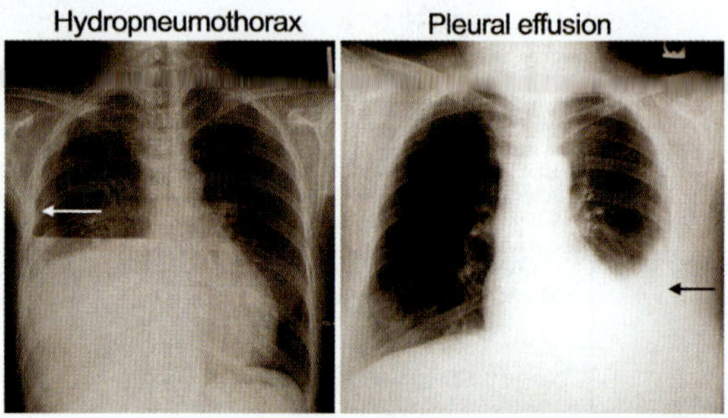

Hampton's hump (pulmonary embolism)

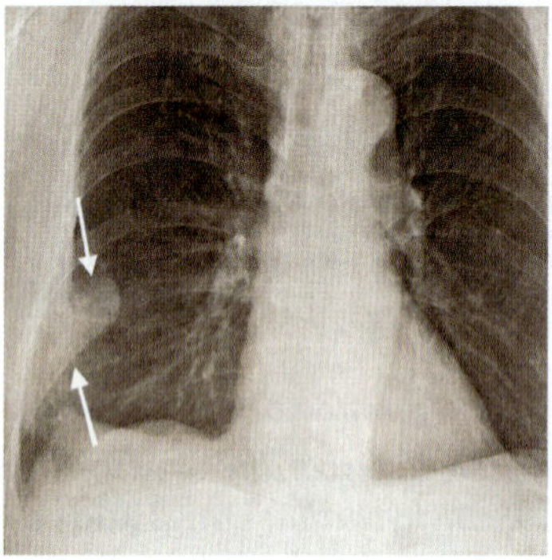

Glasgow coma scale

Observation	*Response*	*Score*
Eyes	Open spontaneously	4
	Open to speech	3
	Open to painful stimulus	2
	No response (no eye opening)	1

Verbal	Responds sensibly	5
	Confused	4
	Inappropriate words	3
	Incomprehensible sounds	2
	No response (silent)	1
Motor	Obeys commands	6
	Points (localizes) to pain	5
	Withdraws from pain	4
	Bend limbs in response to pain (flexion)	3
	Straighten limbs in response to pain (extension)	2
	No response	1

Nexus criteria is used in evaluating a case of suspected C-spine injury

Nexus criteria

1. Absence of tenderness in the posterior midline
2. Absence of a neurological deficit
3. Normal level of alertness (GCS score = 15)
4. No evidence of intoxication (drugs or alcohol)
5. No distracting injury/pain

- Patient who fulfilled all 5 of the criteria were considered low risk for C-spine injury
  - No need C-spine X-ray
- For patients who had any of the 5 criteria
  - Radiographic imaging was indicated (AP, lateral and open mouth views)

Philadelphia hard collar

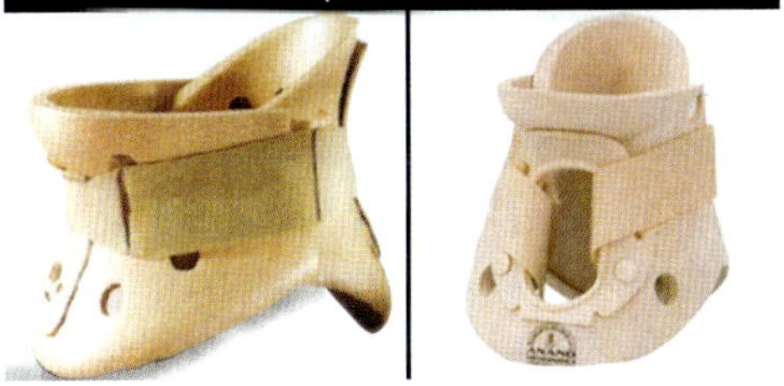

Focussed abdominal sonography in trauma (FAST)

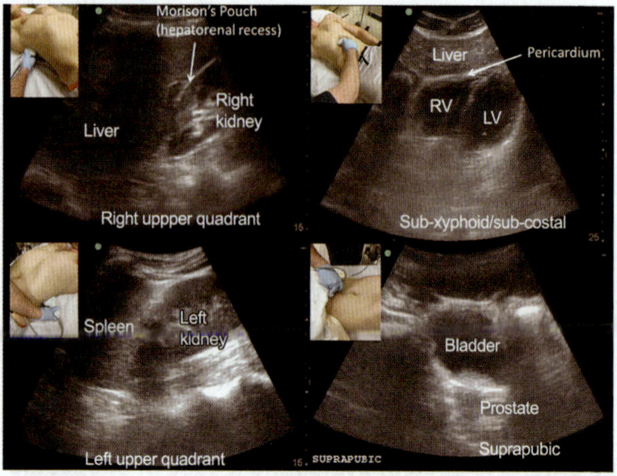

FAST positive

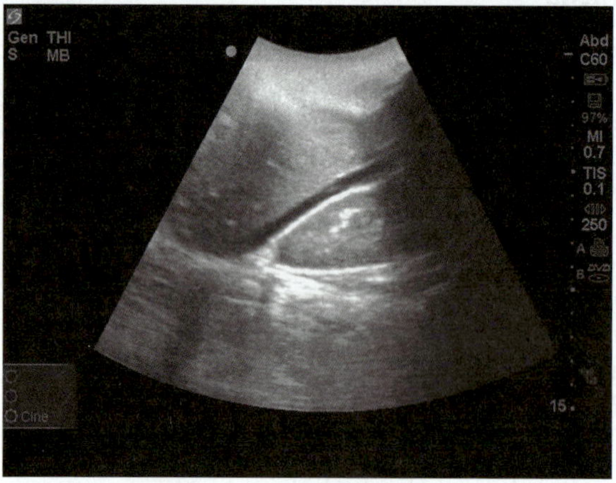

e-FAST (extended FAST)

Includes FAST along with lung ultrasound to detect any life-threatening emergencies like pneumothorax.

Findings in e-FAST

Normal seashore pattern

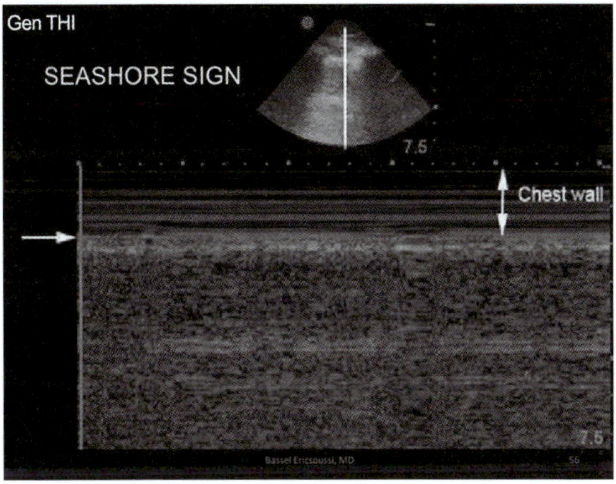

Pneumothorax showing barcode sign

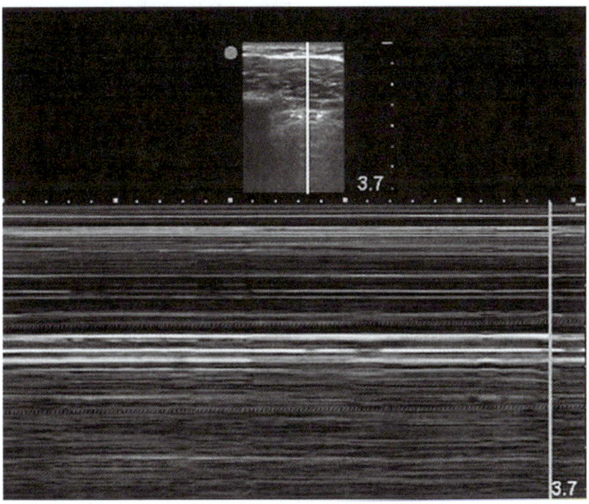